"I can think of no one better qualified to write a book for kidney stone patients than someone who has been a patient herself. Gail Savitz has been through several experiences with stones. In this book, she uses common terms that other patients can understand to explain such things as what lithotripsy means, how stones form, and what you can do to help prevent recurrent stone

—Kenneth

"I reread your chapters in the midst
reassured. What you covered is what most ...
time and volume of information—plus it's much more reassuring to hear about something firsthand. What a treasure this book is for those who need more information."

—Gail Sweeney

"Easy-to-read for patients."

—Urology Times

"The Kidney Stones Handbook is the best! Not a lot of cross talk like most of the others. Straight talk and a true sufferers's perspective."

—Russ Frank

"Thank you again for opening my eyes, and giving me some hope that I thought I would never find again."

—Lisa D.

"I congratulate you on an excellent text. It contains a wealth of information, not only for the patient, but also, I suspect, for the physician and the research scientist. Certainly from my own point of view, there's much in your book that is of great interest to me and which I was not aware of."

—Allen L. Rodgers, Ph.D.
Department of Chemistry
University of Cape Town, South Africa

"This book would be especially worthwhile for the patient with recurrent stone disease who is motivated to fully participate in the prevention of further stone development."

—Urologic Nursing

"I highly recommend this book to urologists, endocrinologists, family practitioners, and their patients."

—SEDMS Medical Librarian

"This book is packed with information to help those who suffer from kidney stones, and to educate the health professionals who treat them. From a librarian's standpoint however, the most valuable section is Chapter 28—the references. You have done an outstanding job of listing additional information resources, books and even a web site for further study on the topic. I refer patients and physicians to it frequently."

—Dorothy Thurmond, MLS
Sutter Hospital
Roseville, CA

"This is an outstanding book that I have enjoyed reading. It provides an enormous amount of information for patients with nephrolithiasis problems. Congratulations."

—Dean Assimos, M.D.
Professor of Urology
Wake Forest University
School of Medicine

"You have outdone yourself once again. I can see that you have added some valuable new information."

—Ross Holmes, Ph. D.
Director of Urology Research
Wake Forest University
School of Medicine

"Because of the dual perspective from patient and urologist, this book by Gail Savitz and Stephen W. Leslie, M.D. provides patients with 'both sides of the coin.' This clear, patient-friendly, illustrated book ends with a glossary and educational resources available to the patient."

—Family Urology
Volume V. Issue 1
American Foundation for Urologic Disease

The
KIDNEY
STONES
Handbook

A Patient's Guide to Hope, Cure and Prevention

Gail Savitz
Stephen W. Leslie, M.D.

Foreword by Martin I. Resnick, M.D.

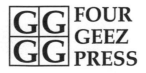

FOUR
GEEZ
PRESS

Roseville, CA

The Kidney Stone Handbook: A Patient's Guide to Hope, Cure and Prevention. Copyright ©1999 by Gail R. Savitz. Printed and bound in the United States of America. All rights reserved. No part of this book may be reproduced in any form or by electronic or mechanical means including information storage and retrieval systems without permission in writing from the publisher, except by a reviewer, who may quote brief passages in a review. Published by Four Geez Press, PMB 131, 1911 Douglas Blvd, Suite 85, Roseville, CA 95661.

Second Edition

Second Printing August 2000
ISBN 0-9637068-6-1

Cover design by Grant W. Gibbs

Four Geez Press participates in the Cataloging in Publication program of the Library of Congress. However, in our opinion, the data provided us for this book by CIP does not adequately nor accurately reflect its scope and content. Therefore, we are offering our librarian/users the choice between LC's treatment and our Alternative CIP.

Publisher's Cataloging in Publication

Savitz, Gail R. and Stephen W. Leslie, M.D.
The Kidney Stones Handbook: A Patient's Guide to Hope, Cure and Prevention
p. cm
Includes medication list and index
ISBN 0-9637068-6-1

1. Kidney 2. Medical Care-United States 3. Diseases related to kidney stones 4. Medical Research 5. Consumer Education 6. Stone Prevention 7. Lithotripsy 8. Diet Related to Kidney Stones 9. Urolithiasis

RC916.G65 1999   616.622

Library of Congress Cataloging-in-Publication Data
(Prepared by Quality Books Inc.)

Savitz, Gail R. and Stephen W. Leslie, M.D.
The Kidney Stones Handbook: A Patient's Guide to Hope,
 Cure and Prevention /
p. cm.
Includes medication list and index.
ISBN 0-9637068-0-1

1. kidney—Calculi—Popular works   I. Title

RC916.G65 1999   616.622
                    QB193-1102

Printed in the United States of America

Dedication

This book is dedicated
to Jerry Barfield,
whose love has internationally helped kidney stone patients
and
Dolores Gibbs-Chamberlain,
a faithful sister who didn't know what questions to ask

Acknowledgements

I would like to thank the following people who took the time to assist me with their invaluable talent in producing this book: David Cohler, editor; K.D. Profitt, Medical Librarian, Sutter Resource Library, Sutter Hospitals; Dorothy Thurmond, Medical Librarian, MLS, Sutter Roseville Medical Center; Robert Downing, photographer; Bob Smith, Auburn, California; Mark Stivers, Sacramento News & Review; Audrey Scannell; Bettina Flores, author of "Chiquita's Cocoon," and "The Millionairess Across the Street;" Rosemarie Emerson, Law Librarian; Ruth Letner; Colleen Nihen, Right Angle Productions, Roseville, California; Mark S. Samberg, M.D., urologist; Alex M. Blaine, Blaine Company Inc., Pharmaceuticals; Kenneth B. Woods, M.D., urologist; Gail Sweeney, Pacific Grove, California; Debby Switters, R.N., American Urological Association Allied; Larrian Gillespie, M.D.; Dr. Ross Holmes; Dr. Allen Rodgers; Dean Assimos, M.D. urologist; Myrna Fox; my daughter Jennifer Golomb; Grant Gibbs my friend, mentor and love; and Bart the Basset who spent many hours sitting at my feet.

And on behalf of Dr. Stephen W. Leslie: to my wife Rosemary I. Moroni, MD, for her understanding and loving patience; and to my patients who ask wonderful questions and support my various projects which tend to keep me tied to the computer.

Table of Contents

Foreword

Kidney stones are a common problem. Estimates indicate that 15 percent of the population will form a stone some time during their life and many of these patients will also go on to form recurrent stones as well. It is also recognized that due to the cost of evaluation and treatment that significant healthcare dollars are expended for this disorder. Finally, and unfortunately, proper evaluation of patients with kidney stones is often not undertaken for it is well recognized that recurrent disease can often be prevented or reduced with proper dietary/medical intervention.

The Kidney Stones Handbook: A Patient's Guide to Hope, Cure and Prevention addresses the problem of kidney stone disease. In a simple and straightforward manner, the authors review the causes and types of stones, the evaluation that is necessary and outline methods of treatment and prevention. In that many years ago many patients required operations to remove stones, today fragmentation and removal can be accomplished with minimal intervention. Though only few stones can be dissolved, many can be prevented with appropriate diet and medications. These aspects of the disorder are reviewed by the authors.

Many handbooks are available today which are written for patients with many different disorders. The current book is unique for its depiction of kidney stone disease. All patients who either have formed kidney stones or are prone to them because of family history or lifestyle pattern should find it of interest and of value.

Martin I. Resnick, M.D.
Lester Persky Professor Chairman
Department of Urology
Case Western Reserve University
University Hospitals of Cleveland
Cleveland, Ohio

Talk Me Through The Hard Times Ahead

Dear Gail:

Hello. My name is Lisa. I am 25 years old. I have been a kidney stone sufferer for the past 13 years. In February, my doctor found four stones in my left kidney. In August, I had lithotripsy. A few weeks later, I found through X-rays only one of the four stones had been broken into small enough pieces to pass. It took me six weeks to pass stone fragments from only one stone.

In September, I was treated again with lithotripsy. Five days later, I went to the doctor to have X-rays. I was told that one of the three stones had broken very well; the last stone, well, had been knocked out of the kidney into the ureter. It is stuck for now.

What I am asking of you is your help. I need to be able to talk with someone who knows how it really feels to hurt so bad that you just want to die. Please give me someone to talk to who is also a sufferer of such pain and discomfort. I have been dealing with this set of stones as well as the pain for seven long months. I have a wonderful husband who tries to help me get through all of this, but as you know, if you have never been through it, you don't really understand. That's why I am writing you, to ask you to please help me, and talk me through the hard times ahead of me.

Lisa

INTRODUCTION

Why I Rewrote This Book
by Gail Savitz

When the first edition of "The Kidney Stones Handbook: A Patient's Guide to Hope, Cure and Prevention" was published in 1994, it was the only book written specifically for patients with stones. Accurate and reliable information about preventing kidney stones was difficult to find and usually written in highly technical language even some doctors couldn't easily make out. My goal was to write a book in plain English that everyone could understand which would give every kidney stone sufferer important information about what was happening to them and emphasize how to minimize their chances of making new stones.

The book was very successful and sold out in record time with little more than word-of-mouth advertising. It was recommended by many fine doctors including former Surgeon General C. Everett Koop, M.D. The goal for this new edition is the same, but there is so much new information that needed to be added that the book was totally rewritten!

A kidney stone sufferer wrote to me asking if this new edition would help her learn more about kidney stone prevention when she already owned the first edition. She asked me, "How will your new book differ from the first one?"

A fair question—and the answer is, not only has medicine changed, *I've changed.*

First of all, as an author and patient, I've altered my attitude since writing the first edition. In the five years since its publication, I've had it up to here (she points to the top of her head) with physicians who allow their patients to become repeat stone formers, who do not provide their patients with lists of foods high (and low) in oxalates, who do not perform metabolic stone risk tests on their patients, who practice without a medical diagnosis, who don't inform their patients about specific medications to prevent stone recurrence, and, yes, with patients who fail to comply with proven methods which can prevent stones in up to 98 percent of all patients.

This second edition is the result of five additional years of research, study, and professional relationships with stone prevention medical experts from around the world. I've been in touch with thousands of kidney stone patients, and I am just now hearing from many patients who bought the first book and who are living life stone free.

I attended my second American Urological Association (AUA) convention in Dallas, Texas where it seemed that "Viagra" was more important and sensational than kidney stone prevention. While impotence and kidney stones are both medical issues which affect the quality of life, I walked away feeling that to some in the AUA, kidney stone patients were stepchildren. We don't complain loudly enough and we routinely accept the most extreme form of cruelty: severe, avoidable, recurrent physical pain.

While not included in the Top Ten Glamour Disease-of-The-Month Club, kidney stone disease still affects over 1.2 million additional people a year with excruciating and debilitating pain, is frequently preventable and poorly understood by most patients, their families and even many physicians.

I write a patient education newsletter on kidney stones. I believe one hundred percent in what I'm doing and I'm not afraid to tell patients that they have been the victims of medical mismanagement, neglect and ignorance when it comes to preventing their stones. To be fair, I don't usually hear from patients who found good doctors who've emphasized stone prevention techniques and helped them with understandable expert advice, testing and treatment. If you are lucky enough to have found such a physician with a genuine interest and expertise in stone prevention, please call or write me with your doctor's name, address and phone number so I can refer other patients.

This book is also different because I've become the first "official" kidney stone patient advocate in the United States! This is the only book written by both a kidney stone patient and stone prevention medical specialist. While I'm not a physician, I go to bat for "my" patients. I treat my book buyers like family. I refer them to stone prevention medical experts. I answer their questions. And if I don't know the answer, I'll find a medical expert who does. I am a library as well. I offer a virtual resource center if you visit my web site at http://www.readersndex.com/fourgeez. From that web site, you can access many medical articles on stone disease written by the nation's top stone prevention doctors and researchers. You can ask questions and request reprints of specific articles written just for us on topics of interest to most stone formers.

If you've had one kidney stone, you don't ever want to repeat that horrendously painful experience! The reality is that about 12 percent of all adult Americans will have a kidney stone at some point in their lives. While women run less risk than men, their chances of forming stones has risen along with their increasing life expectance and generally improved socio-economic status.

Stones tend to run in families. If one family member has a stone, then the risk of another related family member developing a stone increased by an average of 62 percent! The likelihood of a person eventually forming a stone if his brother already had one is 50 percent. If even one parent had a kidney stone, then the risk of stones forming in their children doubles. Although there may be a familial tendency to form stones, the fact that your parents or siblings had them is by no means a guarantee that you will. You can take charge of your life and reduce your risk through education and knowledge. This book gives you that opportunity.

So why did I really write this book? I couldn't enjoy my life waiting for and worrying about the kidney stone pain that could (and would) return at any time. I was sick and tired of becoming another statistic! With each visit to the emergency room, I felt as if I were giving birth to glass shards through my urinary tract! And for months I passed stone after stone after stone. I became absolutely determined to find out how to stop making kidney stones. I wanted to learn as much as possible about them. My life became a quest for this knowledge. This book is the end result of that long quest to find answers about kidney stone formation, treatment and prevention. I just couldn't bear to watch others go through the same pain I had without trying my best to help them by sharing this vital information.

Desperate parents have stood at my front door pleading for a copy of the book "to end the misery"of their children. Some sufferers wanted copies sent overnight at rates twice the book's list price. I still receive some of the most heart-wrenching, personal correspondence from patients who need answers, who are afraid, who do not know what to expect and who are exasperated with repeated surgical and lithotripsy procedures because they continue to pump out one stone after another with little effort or investigation into the cause of their stones or how to prevent them.

Even though kidney stone attacks are possibly the most painful of all human conditions and patients continue to be classified as medical insurance risks, prevention is possible and highly successful with sophisticated medical testing and specific treatment. It's also quite cost effective. For example, the cost for each extracorporeal shock wave lithotripsy (stone fragmentation treatment) is about $7,500 while the average annual net cost savings for patients with active stone disease who have complete metabolic testing including all the extra doctor's visits, medications and supplements is over $2,000 per year. Yet despite the proven cost savings involved, most health insurance companies are reluctant to promote true kidney stone prevention programs although most will cover if ordered by your physician.

As mentioned earlier, every year more than 1.2 million Americans will develop a kidney stone and the number is steadily increasing. More patients make kidney stones than those who suffer strokes each year (400,000 - American Academy of Neurology); more than the 36,000 Americans who develop brain tumors yearly (American Brain Tumor Association) and the 250,000 Americans who suffer from multiple sclerosis (National Multiple Sclerosis Society). Yet, very few doctors or anyone else write about preventing kidney stones in language easily understood by their patients, their partners and families.

While a lot of good information is found on the Internet, most of it is not based on any formal studies or research. Some of it perpetuates myths and misconceptions regarding stone formation; most is based on personal experience and lacks medical references and authorities. The information in this book is supported by scientific fact, including the most recent medical studies, articles and research.

Now, more than nine years after my last stone attack, my struggle continues as I fight, and so far, succeed in preventing any new stones from forming. After extensive research in countless medical and public libraries and with the advice and help of stone prevention medical practitioners and researchers throughout the world, I am now able to offer this completely rewritten "Kidney Stones Handbook: A Patient's Guide to Hope, Cure and Prevention." Thus, from a small nugget of information prior to the book's first publication in 1994 has grown this ultimate guide and resource for stone patients, their families and even the medical professionals who take care of us.

Over the last 16 years, dramatic advances in medical knowledge and research have improved the quality of care possible for people with kidney stones. **There is no valid reason for any patient with the strong desire to prevent future stone attacks to be denied the opportunity.**

If you have already formed a kidney stone, the following chapters will detail the treatments available to get rid of the stone, the causes for each stone type and encouraging news on the latest medical advances in preventing repeat episodes of those terribly painful little pebbles.

Detailed nutrition charts and other resources are among the unique aspects of this book and are included to assist you in choosing foods which will not predispose you to forming new stones. Carry this book with you when you shop for groceries and choose from among a wide variety of foods which can be enjoyed for optimum health and minimum stones.

This book represents a team effort among the most respected and educated medical professionals in the field of kidney stone treatment and prevention. We know your pain. We know your exasperation and fear. Our goal is to guide you through your stone experience and help you prevent future stones.

We wanted to provide you with the most complete patient information on kidney stones that exists to date. We believe we have succeeded.

One of the most significant changes from the first edition that I've taken on a co-author. He is Stephen W. Leslie, M.D., an outstanding stone prevention urologist who lives and

breathes patient education and who is one of the most knowledgeable and dedicated stone prevention experts I've met.
He's a great teacher and a pretty good writer which is a rare
combination to find! He is also a most compassionate fellow,
as well.

So with this edition, I'd like to introduce you to a good
friend of mine, Stephen W. Leslie, M.D.

Why I Helped Co-Author This Book

by Stephen W. Leslie, M.D.

When I read the first edition of "The Kidney Stones Handbook: A Patient's Guide to Hope, Cure and Prevention," I was very surprised to see it written by a patient. My first impression was to call the author to express my outrage at being left out since the stone prevention laboratory protocol I had designed was not included. Little did I know that Gail Savitz would eventually ask me to co-author the new book. In Gail I found a kindred spirit, someone who felt as passionately as I did about bringing kidney stone prevention information directly to the millions of patients who suffer from this terribly painful affliction.

I never expected that treating kidney stone disease would someday become such a large part of my life. As a urologist, my focus during training had always been on the surgical treatment of kidney stones. Very little instruction was given concerning metabolic testing, analysis, or preventive measures.

When I finished my urology training in 1982, I went to work at a large medical clinic. Being the new guy in town meant that I had plenty of time on my hands while I was getting started. Some of my first patients happened to have kidney stones. After I treated their stones, they actually had the audacity to ask me to help them stop making more! Such impudence! I didn't realize then how little I actually knew about the subject. After all, I had been well trained at two of the very best urology training centers in the country. There wasn't a stone made that I wasn't prepared to treat. I knew all the surgical techniques cold—but I had to start from scratch to learn how to really help my patients stop new stones from forming.

Because I wasn't overly busy during those first few months, I did some library research and starting organizing laboratory protocols to make it easier to gather the necessary information. I questioned my colleagues about kidney stone disease and tried to decipher the complicated and often confusing medical articles written on the subject. Eventually, I came to realize that this was a grossly misunderstood field because of a lack of training in medical school and residency, the high cost and difficulty of obtaining the necessary laboratory studies, and the complicated systems of analysis and interpretation. It's almost as if most of the "experts" had conspired to make the subject of stone prevention as complex as possible to enable only a relatively few doctors to offer the service. I decided to try and make it simple by using a sophisticated "expert" computerized analysis so any physician who wanted it could get a complete evaluation of a patient at a reasonable price, along with a written summary of the conclusions and possible preventive therapies.

Ten years ago, this program became commercially available through Roche Biomedical Laboratories (now Laboratory Corporation of America, or "LabCorp") and won the prestigious Thirlby Award of the American Urological Association.

Despite the program's availability, most patients were still not getting this prevention testing or treatment. Some of my urology colleagues actually told me they were not interested in preventing kidney stones because they would not be doing as much surgery and would lose money!

Eventually it became clear that the only way to force some of my reluctant medical colleagues to emphasize kidney stone prevention was to go over their heads and educate their patients. Imagine, educating patients! Revolutionary! And if enough patients demanded stone prevention testing and treatment from their physicians, we would soon find a way to accommodate them.

We now know that we can find treatable causes for kidney stones if we look hard enough. It has also been shown that virtually every patient who follows treatment based on appropriate testing, proper interpretation, and sound medical principles will substantially reduce or eliminate all future kidney stone production. If your doctor doesn't advise such testing in your case, ask him or her about it — and, if necessary, be prepared to demand it.

That's why I decided to help Gail revise and update this new edition.

Stephen W. Leslie, MD FACS
Assistant Clinical Professor
Department of Urology
Medical College of Ohio

Founder and Medical Director
Lorain Stone Research Center
771 West 38th Street
Lorain, Ohio 44052

CHAPTER ONE

The Pebble That Hurts

The sudden wave after wave of searing, ripping pain from an unexpected kidney stone knocked the wind out of me.

It was the kind of pain I would soon learn that some emergency room nurses tell their patients, both male and female, "you are now going through labor pains with this one!"

I could handle two caesarean births, but the pain of a kidney stone was the worst pain I'd ever felt.

A stone that forms in the kidneys and blocks the urinary tract is probably the single most painful disorder to afflict human beings.

Only a few hours earlier, I thought I was developing a bladder infection (although I had not had one in a decade). I was not ready for the hot, knife-like, wrenching pain that continued to slash through my left side, migrating down into my lower abdomen. I thought if I could lie down on a heating pad and not move at all, the pain would diminish.

In addition to the pain came round after round of nausea. I became "addicted" to the toilet while vomiting, and within a short time, I felt extremely dehydrated. Along with the sudden onset of pain up and down my left side, I felt my bladder spasm with painful cramping and yet I was unable to urinate.

> I didn't know whether to stand up, sit down, lie down, or die.
>
> **Gail Savitz, author**

My primary care physician's office would not open for another two hours. Should I go to the emergency room? I decided to wait and see.

As I counted out those endless minutes on that cool summer morning, I had become a new statistic: I was now one of more than 1.2 million Americans who would develop a kidney stone in any given year, and more than 30 million over a lifetime.

Most of these stones range in size from a pencil point to the size of a golf ball and can cause agonizing pain in the lower abdomen and back.

I should have gone to a hospital emergency room immediately. This was a new experience and I tried so valiantly to play down the severe pain I was feeling. It was all in my head, right?

And who would step in and take care of my own children who were sound asleep in the early morning?

A patient can expect a small amount of blood in the urine from minor trauma caused by the stone.

When should a person call the doctor?

Call your doctor or go to the emergency room if you experience:

- Severe pain not controlled by oral pain medication.
- Fever
- Visible blood or clots in the urine
- Persistent vomiting.
- Inability to take oral fluids.
- Severe or persistent diarrhea.
- You have a history of a solitary kidney, renal failure or are currently pregnant.

You can not make the diagnosis of kidney stones yourself. Even if you're sure the pain is identical to your last stone attack, you could be wrong and have to suffer the consequences if it just happens to be your appendix.

As the family's breadwinner, I had no time, nor patience to become ill. I was a single mother with two children and I did not want to scare them. I thought the pain was "all in my head" and I really wasn't as sick as I felt.

What I didn't know was that I had embarked on a journey of cold fear, obnoxious pain, high medical expenses that would leave me strapped financially, unknown procedures and tests that left me terrified with very little knowledge or understanding about the "pebble" that hurt so much.

It was a journey that began with no control over my health. It seemed that my body had become my enemy. After extensive research in countless medical and public libraries, I have begun to understand kidney stone disease. I am able to ask my urologist "intelligent" questions and I feel fortunate to have found a physician who is willing to take the time to answer them all. As I began my own medical research, I realized the information I collected would benefit other patients with kidney stones. Thus, from a seedling of information grew a book for all kidney stone patients.

Kidney stones are a life-long ailment. If you have kidney stones, or you know someone who does, or there is a family history of kidney stones, then this book is for you.

Tales of Torture: My First Kidney Stone

I had been sitting quietly at my computer editing a client's book on parenting. I enjoyed working in the early morning hours before my children, Gary, who was then 12 years old, and Jennifer, then 9 years old, awoke.

When the first kidney stone made its torturous journey down my ureter, I had two health-care options. I could use the large health maintenance organization under which I had health insurance, or consult with the friendly, young physician who had gotten to know me well over the past seven years but whom I would have to pay entirely out of my own pocket.

At that moment of ultimate agony, money had no meaning for me. I would go to whichever medical office answered the phone first.

I desperately tried to get through to the HMO's phones that morning. I kept getting a busy signal. My pain was too intense (and I had no patience under those conditions) to keep trying the appointment line, so I called my internist. They booked an appointment for me within the hour.

While I was in no shape to drive a car that morning, I made an unwise decision to drive. I took my son along as my "comfort blanket." He was completely bewildered and scared by my pain, and there was little that he could do other than be there for me. Each bump in the road was like a sword through my side. Both of my children were scared that I was going to die. It was equally difficult to leave little Jennifer home alone.

My physician immediately took an office X-ray. It was the first of hundreds more to come over the years. When he came back into my examining room, he told me I was passing a kidney stone.

At that moment, it was the worst news he could have given me.

Visions of My Mother

His news that I had a kidney stone upset me greatly. Not only did my mother have kidney stones, but also my paternal grandmother. And my brother has passed two or more kidney stones in a single month!

I remembered how as a young girl I had watched my mother endure horrendous pain with her own kidney stones. Growing up, I saw the long scars on her back from kidney surgery. I remembered how much I missed her when she was hospitalized.

I grew up fearing my mother's pain without understanding it.

Finally, at age 38, I was horrified to be told (in my own heightened state of anxiety) that my mother's pain had become mine as well.

According to the National Institutes of Health (NIH), in the past it was true that little could be done for most patients with stones. "With a surprising lack of fanfare," wrote a noted scientist recently, "recurrent renal stones have become a preventable disease."

There was existing treatment for some of the rarer forms of stones, but patients with the most common kinds of kidney stones faced the prospect of drinking a lot of liquids and the likelihood of surgery. They were told to avoid calcium in their diets. Not until the mid-1990's did researchers realize that for many stone sufferers, lack of calcium in the diet actually contributed to stone formation!

What I did not know the day my first stone hit me was how far medical science had progressed since my mother's own fight with kidney stones with advances in diagnostic X-ray techniques, non-invasive surgical treatment, risk factor analysis and new preventive care over the "stone age" medical management she had received some 35-years earlier.

Today, scientific progress has brought greater understanding of the causes and mechanisms of stone formation and far more effective clinical management of stone disease.

My internist told me that my kidney stone, due to its size, could become a life-threatening situation. He told me that it was important I go back to my HMO and demand the care I desperately needed, along with additional medical tests to fully evaluate and hopefully prevent future stones.

"If you can't find someone to drive you, we'll need to call an ambulance for you," my doctor told me.

Learning to Ask for Help

While I didn't want an ambulance, I also didn't want to disturb any of my friends who were working. I didn't think it was fair to take them away from paying jobs on my behalf.

This attitude was one I learned to change. Over the next three years, I learned to ask for help when I needed it. I got tired of leaving my car in the hospital parking lot when I was admitted as a patient, and asking other people to drive my car home for me.

Instead, I learned to ask friends to spend the night with my two children, and I learned that sometimes it was necessary to call a friend in the middle of the night for a ride to the emergency room. People were more than willing to lend a hand to help.

A nurse called a friend for me. During the hour I waited for him to arrive, my doctor administered two shots for pain and I settled down on his examining table. At long last, I was able to lie down and relax. The pain medication made me less nauseous and the hot, knife-like pain in my back subsided until I arrived at the hospital.

My friend decided to drop off Gary at home before taking me to the hospital. I tried lying down in the back seat of the car and during the entire trip I vomited continuously into a plastic garbage can liner.

Symptoms of Stones

Some people have "silent" kidney stones which produce no discomfort. But most stones cause pain so severe that it's unforgettable. The pain may come in waves that begin in the lower back and move to the side or groin.

Most people can correctly identify the exact site of their stone just by pointing to where the pain is worst.

The severe, constant pain continues as the muscles in the walls of the blocked ureter try to squeeze the stone along into the bladder. The pain is unrelated to the size of the stone and is not caused by the stone "moving" or scratching as many people believe. In fact, the pain is caused by the dilating or stretching and cramping caused by the blockage the stone produces when it gets stuck in the ureter. (The ureter is the muscular tube that drains urine from the kidneys into the urinary bladder).

When the urine produced by the kidney cannot pass the blockage, the ureter and urinary system stretch. The ureter is composed of muscles and will contract or cramp when stretched. This stretching, dilating and cramping is what causes the intense pain.

This also explains why the stones usually don't cause pain when they are just sitting inside the kidney. Since they don't produce any blockage, stretching or dilating of the urinary system, they don't usually produce any pain until they pass out of the kidney and get stuck. The degree of pain is unrelated to the size of the stone, so it's possible to have excruciating pain from a stone smaller than a grain of rice.

Sometimes the patient will find blood in the urine, and may experience a burning sensation during urination, or frequency of urination.

Other symptoms of stones include nausea, the presence of urinary infection accompanied by fever, vomiting, loss of appetite, and chills. The patient may find that his kidney and abdomen in the region of the stone are very tender to the touch.

At the hospital, my friend gave the receptionist my medical information. I spent most of the time vomiting in the restroom. When I returned to the waiting area, there was a wheelchair waiting for me. The severe pain, however, prevented me from relaxing long enough to sit in the wheelchair for any length of time.

The Emergency Room

While standing up against the hospital's wall, I noticed how cool it felt against my hot back. For the next 40 minutes, until I was taken into the emergency room, I virtually climbed the wall with my back. I am sure others in the emergency room found my antics humorous; for me, the wall's coolness seemed to help me tolerate the pain.

When my name was finally called I was led to a gurney. The gurney became my cocoon for the next fourteen hours. I arrived at the hospital during the cool summer morning hours and would leave after darkness had enveloped the river city called Sacramento, California.

The hospital first placed a white patient identification band around my left wrist. From that moment on, I knew I was in serious trouble.

I was given intravenous pain medication (medication that is injected into a vein) and saline solution to replace nutrients lost from vomiting. I could absorb fluids through the IV hookup, but I was given nothing to drink in case I required emergency surgery.

I began to feel the pain medication as it worked its way, first through my lower back, and then as it settled into my shoulders. Within minutes, the pain from the stone was nearly gone. I thought it was possible at that moment that life could continue—maybe.

The IV needle would be helpful as the day progressed and other tests were taken.

The emergency room physicians led me through a maze of tests in order to perform a medical evaluation. It was important they find out exactly where the stone was, its size, shape, and determine what kind it was in order to plan any further treatment.

If the stone was too large to pass, I would require surgery. If it was not life-threatening I could undergo, at a later date, a new stone-crushing method called lithotripsy (ESWL). In some cases, special medications, depending on the type of stone involved, might dissolve the stone.

The X-ray taken in the physician's office had established the presence of a stone. The emergency room physicians, however, performed a quick analyses of my blood and urine to help determine the cause (if any) of this crisis, identify any infections and to plan the proper course of treatment.

More X-rays were taken of the stone.

In most cases, if the stone is small the patient usually needs only pain relief and instructions concerning recovery of the stone after it is passed. If the stone is smaller than 5 mm or about 1/4 inch in diameter, then it will probably pass without surgery. If the stone is greater than 10 mm or about 1/2 inch in width, then it almost certainly will not pass. Whenever possible, urologists usually like to give the stone every chance to pass without resorting to surgery (see page 159).

Whether one is at home or in an emergency room, it is important to "catch" the stone. "Stone catchers," usually cone-shaped cups with cotton or mesh-like filters, are used to help strain the urine. The patient urinates through these cups and, with luck, the stone will be found lying on the filter's bottom. (I have often felt like an early gold miner looking for treasure at the bottom of the pan!). Paint strainers also work, but my favorite stone catcher is an aquarium net usually used for goldfish.

A year later during another kidney stone crisis, the stone snagged itself on my skin as I went to the bathroom and I was able to retrieve it with toilet tissue. It's sharp-sided edge felt like a rose thorn.

Sometimes in a busy emergency room, a nurse may forget to give the patient a cup, or stone catcher, in which to catch the kidney stone. This has happened to me on two different occasions, and the stone was never found. It is very important that patients ask for this mesh-like strainer before they empty their bladders.

Catching the stone helps the physician determine treatment and develop a prevention program. A chemical stone analysis may suggest the cause of the stone by identifying its composition.

Every patient with a possible kidney stone will require some type of imaging study of the urinary tract. The most common forms of imaging are ultrasound, intravenous pyelogram (IVP), retrograde pyelograms and computerized tomography (CT) scans. Other studies, such as a single flat X-ray of the abdomen (called a "KUB" for kidney, ureter and bladder) and especially plain tomograms of the kidneys are useful in following the progress of the stone disease. (These will be reviewed in a later chapter.)

A patient's first IVP can be a frightening experience. However, I have found that helpful technicians or physicians who have administered the IVP while standing next to the patient can reassure an anxious stone sufferer by explaining the procedure and what to expect.

The IVP has been the gold standard for diagnosis of kidney stones for many years. It is now being replaced in many institutions by CT scans which are faster, safer, and more likely to help make a diagnosis if a stone is not present.

I felt the IVP solution travel through my vein. It felt cold at first, and within a few minutes I could feel a metallic taste in my mouth. The physician stayed with me and told me what I might expect. This lessened my fear and anxiety.

Once the dye was administered, X-rays were taken which highlighted the kidneys and ureters as well as the bladder.

During the day and into the early evening hours, I was given a lot of pain medication. It made me dizzy and disoriented, but those feelings were better than managing a stone without any pain medication.

At long last, I was discharged from the emergency room. While I had passed the stone during my time in the emergency room (subsequent X-rays showed the stone was gone), I did not "catch" it.

Instead, I was given the next worst kind of news: there was a second, much larger stone in my kidney (the left one).

In my hand, I clutched both a prescription for pain medication and an appointment slip for a follow-up visit with a new urologist. I was taking my first step on a long journey to understanding what had happened to me and what, if anything, I could do to prevent this day from ever happening again.

What I didn't know was that I would be hospitalized twice again, pass three more large kidney stones, undergo lithotripsy (ESWL) three times, and greet the future; a future I could survive with proper nutrition, adequate fluids, and prescription medications, thanks to some of the sophisticated medical advances now available in the management of kidney stones.

CHAPTER TWO

Are You Stone Prone?

During the 1960s, Bob Dylan sang "...everybody must get stoned... Oh, I would not feel so alone; everybody must get stoned."

While Dylan was obviously not singing about kidney stones, just how many people are "getting stoned" yearly with kidney stones?

Over 1.2 million patients each year in the United States produce their first stone and almost 30 million will develop at least one stone at some point in their lives..

People who live near large bodies of water such as an ocean, the Gulf of Mexico, or the Great Lakes tend to have more stones than people living far from water sources. Some countries such as Italy, Israel, Northern Australia, Eastern Europe, Northern India, Pakistan, and Eastern China have a greater incidence of stone disease than the U.S. while Sweden and Japan have a lower rate. People who live in "soft" water areas tend to have more kidney stones than those who live where the water is "hard."

In the U.S., stones occur most frequently in the summer months from June through August. According to the U.S. National Institutes of Health, kidney stones account for about seven to ten out of every 1,000 hospital admissions. One in 10 people is at risk of developing kidney stones at some time. Even more disturbing is the evidence that suggests that the incidence of kidney stones is on the rise. Over a 22-year time span the frequency of kidney stones as a hospital discharge diagnosis increased by 75 percent!

Dr. Lynwood Smith from the Mayo Clinic and a noted kidney stone expert, has written that by the time people in the United States reach age 70, five to fifteen percent will have developed at least one urinary stone.

There is definitely a genetic predisposition to developing kidney stones. If one sibling has a stone, there is a 50 percent chance that each additional sibling will have one at some time. If a parent had a kidney stone, then the chances that a child of theirs will have a stone someday is doubled compared to the general population.

There is a high risk of recurrence in those people with at least one stone episode. Within five years after a first stone, there is a 50 percent chance of another stone attack, assuming no preventive measures are taken. Over 10 years, the risk of yet another stone episode increases to about 75 percent. Some people will be "active" stone formers and show either progressive growth of existing stones or frequent recurrences. About 10 percent of stone formers will be particularly unfortunate and have 10 or more stones in their lifetimes. There are some patients who have averaged one or more stones a month for years before receiving preventive chemical testing (metabolic analysis) and specific stone prevention treatment. The "world record" for the number of stones produced by a single person is well over a thousand!

And there are thousands more patients who make stone after stone without any prevention advice, who never receive the metabolic testing that would identify their chemical risk factors, and who continue to have lithotripsy or other surgeries performed—one after another. We still do not know all the possible long-term effects repeated lithotripsy may have on the human body other than realizing some patients will experience a slight rise in their blood pressure. This will need to be monitored for years to come.

In researching this book, I spoke with a man in his mid-forties who gave up his dream to have a family of his own. A longtime bachelor, he hoped one day to "find the right woman." However, after suffering the immense pain and fear that comes with passing one stone every three months for two decades, he decided to have a vasectomy. He vowed that he would never pass on to his own children an inherited family gene that might condemn them to feel the same pain and hopelessness he had endured.

The peak age for stone disease is usually between 30 and 45 years. The incidence tends to decline over age 50, but those who do form stones in these later years seem to have the same number and types of chemical problems and risk factors as their younger counterparts. Fortunately, preventive testing and specific treatment can help all of these people avoid most recurrences.

What is a Kidney Stone?

A kidney stone is a hardened mineral deposit or concretion that was formed in the kidney (even if it eventually ends up somewhere else in the urinary system). It begins as a microscopic crystal or particle which grows, developing into a collection of crystals and eventually a stone over a period of weeks, months or even years. The most common spot for a stone to form is the area inside the kidney where the renal (kidney) tissue meets the hollow urine drainage system. The lining of the kidney at this border seems to be the ideal place to grow stones.

Kidney stones are always abnormal. They form because of too much or too little of some urinary chemical and not enough water to dissolve all the minerals, compounds and waste products the kidneys are trying to excrete. In other words, kidney stones form when there is just not enough water to dissolve all the materials that the kidneys have filtered from the blood.

For example, if you tried to dissolve a 10 pound bag of sugar in a cup of coffee, you would end up with some slightly wet sugar and a big mess. If you threw that same 10 pound bag into a swimming pool full of water, it would dissolve easily. For the kidneys, this means always having enough water around to easily dissolve any and all chemicals that might come along and need to be excreted. That's why all stone formers are told to drink more water regardless of the type of stone they form. Clearly, they would not have developed that stone if there had been enough water around when the stone was "born" to keep all the minerals and chemicals filtered from the blood by the kidneys in solution and dissolved. At that point, your body just didn't have enough water and a stone was born.

Understanding the Importance of Our Kidneys

Your kidneys are bean-shaped organs, each about the size of your fist. They are located near the middle of your back on either side, just partially behind the rib cage and tucked in under the lungs and diaphragm. Most people, when asked to point to their kidneys, think they're located much lower than they really are.

The kidneys are sophisticated trash collectors. Every day, your kidneys process about 200 quarts of blood to filter out about one and a half quarts of concentrated waste products and excess water. The waste and extra water become urine which flows to your bladder through long muscular tubes called ureters. The ureters can force or pump the urine from your kidneys to the bladder even if you are upside down or weightless in space! Your bladder stores urine until you eliminate it by urination (voiding).

The wastes in your blood come from the normal break-down of body tissues like muscle and from the foods you eat. Your body uses the food for energy, replacement and repair. After your body has taken the food products it needs from the blood, waste is sent back into the bloodstream. If your kidneys did not remove these wastes, they would build up in the blood and damage your body.

Renal Failure (Kidney Failure)

Renal failure is the name of an abnormal condition in which the kidneys are unable to adequately filter the blood and remove the wastes and extra fluid from the body. Artificial kidney machines can remove these wastes through a filtering process called dialysis but there are many problems with this system. Dialysis must be performed regularly to be effective. Problems include blood clotting, weakness, infections and electrolyte abnormalities. Nothing really works as well as your own kidneys. A simple way to estimate kidney function is to measure the blood creatinine level. This protein, called creatinine, is manufactured by the body's muscle tissue at a very regular, predictable rate and is usually filtered easily by healthy kidneys.

When the kidneys lose their filtering ability, the creatinine will build up in the blood and can be measured. It's not dangerous by itself, but it's a useful indicator of kidney function.

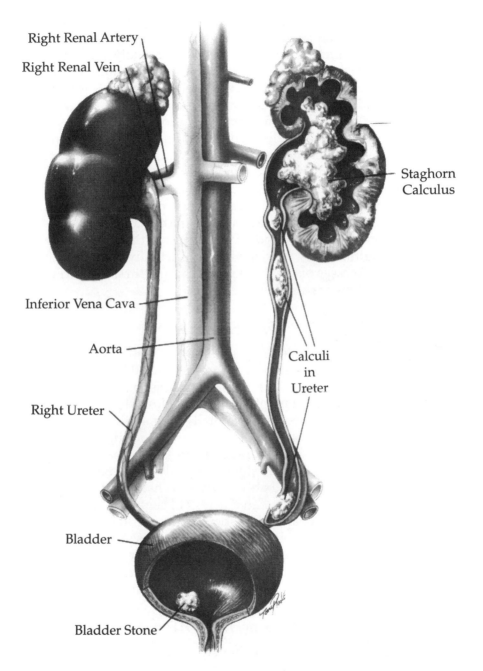

Right Renal Artery

Right Renal Vein

Staghorn
Calculus

Inferior Vena Cava

Aorta

Calculi
in
Ureter

Right Ureter

Bladder

Bladder Stone

Illustration courtesy of Blaine Company Inc., Pharmaceuticals; Erlanger, Kentucky.

The normal range for blood creatinine levels is usually anything up to about 1.5, while potentially dangerous levels of kidney failure would be indicated by a creatinine level of three or more. A blood creatinine of eight, nine or ten would usually indicate complete renal failure and require dialysis.

Kidneys can be damaged permanently by a number of medical conditions such as severe diabetes, various inflammatory and degenerative diseases, genetic disorders, infections, surgeries, injuries and various medications. The Western diet is also suspect as a predisposing factor in the development of renal failure. In particular, a diet containing excessive protein may overly burden the kidneys with digested protein byproducts and wastes.

The kidneys also help control blood pressure, make red blood cells, regulate the salt balance in the blood and keep your bones strong by producing hormones that control these and other functions. (Yes, the kidneys actually make hormones!). In cases of renal or kidney failure, these other regulatory functions are also lost.

Even Mummies Were Stone Prone

The very first known urinary stone was found in an Egyptian mummy, a teenage boy, dating from 4800 BC. It was a bladder stone. Until modern times, the vast majority of urinary stones afflicting mankind were bladder stones. Today, bladder stones that did not originally form in the kidneys are relatively rare in economically developed societies but still fairly common in Third World countries. This change from bladders stones to kidney stones has only occurred since World War II and is probably related to changes in diet.

The mummy's stone had a uric acid center surrounded by layers of calcium oxalate and struvite (infection stone material). In short, a little bit of everything. It was stored in a museum in England until the stone was "pulverized" in 1941, well before lithotripsy had even been invented. (The building it was stored in was bombed during an air raid).

The "Why Me?" Question Often Has Answers

In most cases, you are either stone prone or you're not. A combination of factors causes kidney stones. Physicians have identified several characteristics that appear to increase an individual's chance of developing a kidney stone

The Five Most Common Kidney Stone Chemical Risk Factors:

- Too much urinary calcium (called hypercalciuria)
- Too much urinary oxalate (called hyperoxaluria)
- Too much urinary uric acid (called hyperuricosuria)
- Too little urinary citrate (called hypocitraturia)
- Too little urinary volume and not enough water (called too little urinary volume and not enough water!).

Each of these will be briefly discussed here and in greater detail in subsequent chapters. Additional chemical risk factors include low urinary magnesium, high urinary cystine (a genetic disorder), high urinary sodium and abnormal urinary acid levels.

Various medical conditions can also predispose people to develop stones. These include hyperparathyroidism, renal tubular acidosis, high blood pressure, urinary infections, arthritis, back pain, chronic diarrhea, short bowel syndrome, genetic conditions, endocrine and hormonal disorders, chronic dehydration, urinary tract obstructions and anatomic abnormalities, Crohn's disease, colitis, gout, purine gluttony and loss of beneficial Oxalobacter bacteria from the digestive tract. Any blockage or slowing of the flow of urine also appears to increase the likelihood of kidney stones. All of these are reviewed elsewhere in this book.

Calcium

Calcium helps build strong bones and teeth. It also makes really hard kidney stones! Nearly 85 percent of all stones contain at least some calcium, usually chemically bound to either oxalate or phosphate. (Calcium cannot form a stone unless it is chemically attached to certain other compounds like oxalate and phosphate). Traditionally, most people with calcium stones were told to eat less calcium. Several studies have now proven that this was often exactly the wrong advice! In general, people whose diets include higher amounts of calcium actually tend to have fewer stones. This is because when calcium binds to oxalate in the digestive tract, neither is absorbed or able to form kidney stones. But if the calcium is missing, oxalate will be absorbed at a higher rate and will eventually cause a net increase in calcium stone formation. Just the opposite of what you would expect.

There are several different types of calcium stone problems. One is caused by abnormal hormone levels and can be diagnosed by a simple blood test. Another seems to be due to a kidney defect which allows an excessive amount of calcium to escape into the urine. This "Renal Calcium Leak" problem can be treated very successfully with medications called "thiazides." The most common calcium problem is due to increased absorption of calcium from the diet. This "Increased Intestinal Calcium Absorption" is best treated by dietary calcium moderation plus medication if dietary measures are inadequate.

Being sedentary for any lengthy period of time tends to increase the amount of calcium in the urine and to increase the odds of forming a kidney stone. This is a problem not only for patients confined or convalescing in bed for long periods of time, but also for astronauts in space. Without physical activity to stimulate the bones, calcium tends to leave the bony skeleton and enter the bloodstream where it eventually is filtered out by the kidneys and ends up in the urine. This not only leads to kidney stones, but also weakens the skeleton resulting in brittle bones, fractures and osteoporosis.

Oxalate

Oxalate is an organic chemical that binds strongly to calcium, which is why it forms such hard stones. It is the second most common ingredient in kidney stones next to calcium. As far as we know, oxalate has no significant beneficial function in people, but is both created by the liver as a waste product and absorbed from the diet in roughly equal amounts. Oxalate is primarily found in vegetarian food sources such as green leafy vegetables, teas, some colas, nuts and chocolate. Reductions in dietary oxalate can make a significant difference in stone production. We know that pound for pound, oxalate is about 15 times stronger than calcium as a kidney stone promoter. Various medications can lower urinary oxalate in some people, but there is no single medication currently available that successfully treats this condition in all patients. Combined approaches using both medications and diet are usually required.

New research suggests that the loss of the beneficial ox-
alate-digesting intestinal bacterial called Oxalobacter may be an
important stone promoting factor in some people. More research is needed before this can be confirmed, as well as testing
procedures standardized and specific therapies developed.

Uric Acid

About ten percent of all kidney stones are composed of
uric acid, a substance that also causes gout. Men are more
likely than women to suffer from this type of stone. The bad
news is that uric acid is not visible on standard X-rays. The
good news is that it is the one type of stone that can often be
dissolved with the proper medication. Uric acid is a waste
product primarily of protein digestion. How well it dissolves
in the urine is determined in large part by the overall urinary
acid level. If the urinary acid is a little too high, the uric acid
will not dissolve and can form crystals and stones. One of the
more effective treatments for uric acid stone disease is to use a
measured amount of a urinary antacid such as potassium
citrate on a regular basis.

Low Urinary Citrate

Many of you reading this book will never have heard of
citrate. This very important urinary chemical is second in
importance only to water as a kidney stone inhibitor. In adequate amounts and concentration, it specifically prevents the
formation of calcium oxalate crystals and stones! Citrate is the
kidneys' natural antacid and stone inhibitor. Oral supplements
of potassium citrate can increase the urinary citrate level
substantially. Citrus fruits and lemonade also help, but the
quantity required is usually too great to avoid the need for a
specific corrective citrate supplement.

Certain medical disorders can cause a significant reduction
in urinary citrate levels. For example, renal tubular acidosis is
a medical condition in which the kidneys are unable to excrete
acid, causing it to build up in the body. This creates conditions
inside the kidney that usually lead to the formation of multiple stones. One of the critical diagnostic criteria for this
condition is the finding of extremely low urinary citrate levels.
Potassium citrate supplements can correct many of the ill
effects of this condition and stop the formation of kidney
stones.

Inadequate Fluid Intake

Anything that decreases the amount of fluid in the body, such as low water intake, excessive perspiration or a hot climate may set the stage for kidney stone formation. Various digestive problems including chronic diarrhea, colitis and Crohn's Disease can lead to dehydration and a number of stone producing chemical imbalances as well. If large amounts of water are not replaced quickly enough, the urine will become concentrated with all the urinary waste products that tend to form crystals and stones. Whenever the urine becomes too concentrated, microscopic crystals tend to form, just like ocean water forms salt crystals when the water is allowed to evaporate. Eight glasses of 8 oz. of water each is generally considered an adequate amount to drink on a daily basis for a stone patient. This is very difficult to accomplish for many people. A better solution is to gradually increase the fluid intake by drinking smaller amounts, perhaps only 4 oz. at a time, but more often throughout the day. Eventually your fluid thermostat will "reset" and you'll get thirsty if you cut back on your water intake. The goal is to drink as much as necessary to produce at least two quarts (or more) of urine a day. Without an adequate fluid intake, no amount of dietary or medical therapy is going to succeed in stopping your kidney stone production (see Chapters 14 and 15).

Urinary Tract Infections

Urinary tract infections affect the structure and function of the kidneys and can chemically affect the urine itself leading to stone formation. The most common type of urinary infection is called cystitis which means inflammation of the urinary bladder. This is most prevalent in young women. Untreated urinary tract infections may lead directly to kidney stones known as "struvite" or infection stones. Some infecting bacteria release chemicals that neutralize the acid normally found in the urine. Once this protective acid is gone, the bacteria can grow more quickly. This also leads to chemical changes in the urine which cause the struvite stone material to come out of solution and form stones. Worse, the stones are always infected with the offending bacteria. Without an infection, struvite stones cannot form.

Cystine

Cystinuria, a rare condition in which the presence of excessive amounts of cystine is found in the urine (usually a genetic disorder present since birth) may also contribute to the formation of stones. Cystine is a normal body chemical that is actually an amino acid, one of the essential building blocks of all protein. It doesn't dissolve well in water, but this is not usually a problem since under normal circumstances only a relatively small quantity ever shows up in the urine. Some people are unfortunately born with a congenital or genetic problem with cystine, causing it to be excreted in large amounts in the urine where it forms cystine stones. This type of stone tends to be quite rubbery in texture and is often resistant to lithotripsy. Fortunately, it is a relatively rare disorder. Prevention therapies are available but usually more aggressive, unpleasant and difficult to follow than for the typical calcium stone former.

"New" Stones (Protease Inhibitors)

Chemicals in environmental agents (such as insecticides, solvents, cleaners and other toxic substances) and some medications (like Triamterene, a "water pill") can cause kidney stones.

Recently, a new type of stone, composed of medicines called "protease inhibitors" has developed. Protease inhibitors comprise a group of medications used in the treatment of AIDS. They are currently the most effective drugs available to treat AIDS. The residues of these protease inhibitors are excreted in the urine where they can form stones since they don't dissolve well. The stones are actually composed of the original medicine and its byproducts. The best preventive therapy is to be extra careful to always maintain a high urinary volume if you need to take one of these protease inhibitor medications.

Indinavir sulfate is a powerful protease inhibitor used in the treatment of AIDS. There appears to be a clear association between indinavir sulfate and kidney stone formation. One study reported the results of 183 patients followed for nearly a year and found that an astounding 13.1 percent had symptomatic stones. The researchers looked at 11 patients and 8 of them had radiolucent (meaning the stones don't show up on X-ray) indinavir stones. Non-contrast spiral CT scans are now the initial diagnostic procedure of choice in many emergency rooms across the country. Indinavir stones will not show up on these scans. Instead, a contrast study such as an IVP (Intravenous Pyelogram) or traditional kidney X-rays should be done if a kidney stone is suspected in patients taking protease inhibitor medications. Indinavir stones are vey fragile and usually respond to conservative therapies.

Don't Throw Away Any Stones! (They're Precious!)

The only way your doctor can determine the exact chemical composition of your stone is to make sure that every stone and fragment is collected and analyzed. That is why you *should* always strain all the urine to collect any stones or fragments that might pass for as long as necessary or until your physician tells you to stop. This is the only way to determine for certain what the stone is composed of and how to stop forming more.

While laboratory testing of the blood and urine will show the possible chemical risk factors, only a stone chemical analysis can determine the exact composition. Without both of these results, your doctor can't determine the specific chemical pathway causing your stones. For a complete understanding of your specific stone formation problem and a precise medical diagnosis, your physician needs both the kidney stone chemical composition analysis and the results of a good, complete metabolic stone risk test from a reliable laboratory. (See pages 109 - 100 for a listing of stone prevention testing laboratories.)

Can Vitamin C Make You Stone Prone?

Many people believe that megadoses of Vitamin C can cure everything from the common cold to cancer. But a recent study suggests that the "Wonder Vitamin" may not be so wonderful for people at risk for developing kidney stones. Doses of Vitamin C over 500 mg. per day may put those who are stone prone at risk although the evidence that Vitamin C actually increases stone formation is somewhat conflicting. Theoretically, Vitamin C can be converted by the liver into oxalate which is known to be a strong promoter of kidney stone formation. But does this actually happen?

The prestigious Journal of Urology reported a study in which Dr. Arthur Smith and his team of urologists at Long Island Jewish Medical Center in New York gave 15 patients doses of Vitamin C that ranged from 100 to 2,000 mg. and then checked their urine for oxalate. More oxalate was found in the urine of patients taking 500 mg. or more of Vitamin C. Dr. Smith and his colleagues concluded that doses of Vitamin C greater than 500 mg. are probably not advisable for kidney stone patients.

This study is important because it is safe from the criticism levelled at earlier reports yielding similar results. Vitamin C is known to turn into oxalate when exposed to air and some doctors had argued that previous researchers hadn't taken adequate precautions to preserve the urine which made their results and conclusions suspect. The Long Island Jewish study used patients with urinary catheters placed directly inside their kidneys, thereby significantly reducing the risk of exposure to the air and greatly improving the reliability of their results.

In an editorial, the Journal of Urology suggested that while this one study may not settle the argument about the alleged benefits of Vitamin C supplements, it may at least convince those with a history of calcium oxalate kidney stones to stick to a daily glass of orange juice and just leave it at that!

One patient interviewed for this book, a big, burly home builder who lives in the foothills of the Sierra mountains in California reported that he used to consume large amounts of Vitamin C. "I never had a cold in my life. I had kidney stones—but I never had a cold," he said. "Now, I get colds all the time, but I sure as heck haven't had a stone in 10 years!" he explained.

The Stone-Prone Diet: Your Stone is What You Eat!

Stone researchers have found a number of possible links between diet and stone formation. Data obtained from a variety of economically advanced countries, including Germany and Austria, suggest a very strong correlation between affluence and kidney stones. During the twentieth century in Great Britain, Germany, Italy and Norway the incidence of kidney stone disease was closely associated with political and economic circumstances.

Stone disease has often been linked to a "diet of affluence" because people who can afford to eat more meat in their diets often end up with more kidney stones. Dr. Stanley Goldfarb, a nephrologist from the University of Pennsylvania has suggested that patients with recurrent kidney stones may be more sensitive to the effects of the chemical byproducts found in high animal protein diets. In populations whose intake of dietary meat protein is reduced or absent, such as vegetarians, the risk of kidney stone disease is markedly reduced as long as there isn't an overdose of high oxalate containing fruits and vegetables.

Some studies have suggested that patients with kidney stones adopt a vegetarian diet, even though many vegetables and fruits contain the very substances (oxalates) which form stones. In Great Britain, the prevalence of stone formation was three times less in a group of vegetarians than in the general population. Dr. Goldfarb reported that vegetarians are typically members of the upper social classes in England and the prevalence of stone formation in this group was approximately one eighth of predictions.

Do You Live in The Stone Belt?

In the United States, the "kidney stone belt" is centered in the Carolinas. Surprisingly, Tennessee has the highest reported prevalence of kidney stones of any state. Areas around large bodies of water including the Great Lakes also have a higher incidence. The Northwest, Southeast and Southwest also tend to have more than their fair share of kidney stone patients. Maybe it's the water.

As Dr. Glenn Preminger, urologist at Duke University, said " unless we treat the cause, the patients will form new stones." That's our goal—to treat the cause and stop the madness.

You may indeed be stone prone and have a long family history of stone-plagued relatives; you may also live in a "stone belt" and you may even live near the largest bodies of water in the world—but there is indeed hope and long-term prevention strategies available for you.

If you can't find a doctor who is actively practicing stone prevention, we invite you to contact us for a physician referral.

The patient feedback from our Physician Referral Service shows we have access to some of the most compassionate and knowledgeable stone prevention physicians in the United States. If you're willing to comply with proven methods based on scientific principles and studies, you're a good candidate for stone prevention testing and treatment. Even if the therapy isn't absolutely perfect, you will still make fewer stones than otherwise.

Too many doctors feel kidney stone patients will just not follow stone prevention therapy guidelines. We believe that given a choice, most kidney stone patients would do almost anything to prevent further stone recurrences. The great majority of kidney stone patients are still not given the opportunity to receive metabolic prevention testing and specific prevention therapy.

To contact our Physician Referral Service, or to ask us a questions, our telephoen number is 1-800-2-KIDNEYS.

CHAPTER THREE

There's No Pain
Like Stone Pain

"**O**h, the pain, the agony of it. That man born of woman should suffer so, is an abomination before God! Out, out damned stone! So small a thing, alike in size to a millet seed, to cause such misery as to make the strongest man seem the littlest babe. T'would be a wonder indeed if the misery it made were not so dear. Surely, even the deepest depths of Hell could not approach such torment as this! Would that I would die so the aching would cease. Yea, I would sell my soul for one moments' respite, for to be free of this agony should seem eternal bliss."

Stephen W. Leslie, M.D.
with a nod to Shakespeare

A kidney stone attack is described as the most painful experience possible to live through. It's more painful than gunshot wounds, major surgery, broken bones, burns and even childbirth. Women who have had both childbirth and stones claim that the kidney stone pain was much worse!

Pain Medication

When you hurt, relief is spelled "pain medicine!" This can range from a simple aspirin, Tylenol or Motrin (usually not much help for real stone pain) up to injectable medications used in combination which can control even the worst kidney stone pain.

This section is devoted to a discussion of some of the more commonly used medications that treat kidney stone pain. It's intended to be just a general guideline: to give you an idea of the types of common medicines used for kidney stone attacks. It is not meant to be an extensive or detailed pharmacological review of all the possible drugs and medicines available to treat pain. Other medicines not specifically mentioned here may be chosen by your physicians to help you, but generally they will fall within one of the following categories:

First Line Medications:

These medications are classified as Non-Steroidal Anti-Inflammatory Drugs or "NSAIDS." They all have certain traits in common. They have varying degrees of anti-inflammatory effects and all are reasonably good pain relievers for minor aches and pains but are generally not adequate by themselves for major kidney stone level pain. Aspirin, Aleve, Advil, Motrin and Tylenol would be examples.

Opioids:

Opioid refers to any medication that is chemically related to medicines derived from opium. Opioid medicines work by combining with specific receptors located primarily in the spinal cord and brain. They don't stop the pain from being generated in the body, but they do prevent the brain from receiving the signal and feeling the pain.

All opioid medications have certain traits in common. They all tend to minimize the perception of pain but can also cause drowsiness, constipation, nausea, vomiting, slowing of respirations (breathing) and mood changes. Many people are worried about dependence and possible addiction with these medications. This almost never happens when they are used appropriately for severe pain for limited periods of time of four to six weeks.

There are three chemically distinct categories of opioid medications, but for our purposes there really are only two: oral and injectable.

Oral opioid medications that are taken as pills or tablets would include Codeine, Tylenol with Codeine, Darvon, Darvocet, Vicodin, Lortab, Dilaudid, Percocet and Percodan. They are listed roughly in order of increasing analgesic strength. These medications can be quite effective if the patient is able to take pills at all during a stone attack where nausea and vomiting are common. They are most useful when taken early in a relatively mild stone event and as an alternative to injectable agents whenever possible.

Injectable opioid agents require an intramuscular (IM) or intravenous (IV) injection. Examples would be Morphine and Demerol. (Morphine was named for the Greek God of Dreams, Morpheus). These are very effective pain relieving medicines and can usually stop even severe kidney stone pain depending on the dosages used. Intravenous injections are faster, but also are slightly more risky because of the decrease in breathing rate they can produce. An accidental overdose if given directly into a vein can be very serious. These agents are best used only for very severe pain, switching to oral agents as soon as possible. They can be combined with Toradol (see below) for additional pain relieving effect and with anti-nausea medications to avoid gastrointestinal upset and vomiting.

Injectable Non-Opioid Medications:

In an attempt to find other drugs that would have fewer side effects and less potential for addiction but still possess the excellent pain relieving properties of the opioids, a number of alternative medicines were developed such as Talwin, Stadol and Nubain. This class of drugs is virtually equal to Morphine and Demerol in overall strength (especially Nubain) and do tend to have less side effects and a lower addiction potential. Nubain is probably the most commonly prescribed medicine from this category used for severe kidney stone pain. They should not be used together with an opioid drug because of specific chemical antagonisms between them.

Toradol:

Toradol is a potent analgesic medication that is available both as an injectable agent and a pill. It is not related to the opioid drugs and is actually more similar to aspirin. It works primarily at the site that is actually causing the pain where it reduces or eliminates the pain signal that goes to the brain and spinal cord. It does not have many of the unpleasant side effects of the opioids and will not affect mood or breathing rate. In some people, it is remarkably effective in eliminating even very severe kidney stone pain. In others, less so. It is best used as initial therapy for a severe stone attack or combined with an injectable opioid such as Demerol to eliminate virtually all pain from even the worst kidney stone attacks. When used together, Toradol reduces the pain signal from the site of the stone and Demerol limits the effect this weakened signal has on the pain receptors in the brain and spinal cord.

Anti-Nausea Medications:

Medicines such as Compazine, Phenergan, Reglan and Vistaril will help reduce the nausea and vomiting often associated with kidney stone attacks and the use of injectable Opioid drugs. Several also have a mild tranquilizing effect which is helpful in reducing anxiety, making it easier to control the pain with other agents.

Patient Controlled Analgesia (PCA):

In an ideal world, you would call the nurse when you began to feel the pain returning and they would immediately respond to your request with additional pain medicine delivered instantly. In the real world, it takes time for nurses to finish their work with other patients, notice your call light is on and respond. Then they have to listen to your request, go find the medicine, possibly call the hospital pharmacy to send it up, wait for it, measure it, mix it, prepare and fill the syringe, walk back to your room and finally give you a shot, by which time your discomfort level has climbed up the pain scale to "agony" or worse.

A better way to deliver pain medicine was developed which eliminates the "middleman" and gives you the pain medicine you need instantly. It is called Patient Controlled Analgesia or "PCA."

The "PCA" pump is loaded with pain medicine as selected by your physician. Specific safety limits are set which will not allow the machine to give you too much medication at one time. Whenever you feel you need some additional pain relief, you press a button and the machine immediately delivers a predetermined measured dose of medication directly into a vein where it quickly goes to work relieving your discomfort. Studies have shown that this "PCA" type of delivery system for pain medicine uses substantially less actual medication than standard techniques like injections and most patients prefer it. "PCA" not only eliminates the uncomfortable and unpleasant shots, but you never have to wonder how long it will take to get the pain medicine and relief you need. Just knowing the pain medicine is instantly available makes the whole process less frightening while reducing any anxiety about quickly receiving adequate pain relief.

This "PCA" system may not be ideal in an Emergency Room setting, but if you have to remain in the hospital for a bad kidney stone attack and need injectable pain medication to stay comfortable, be sure to ask your physician to arrange for "PCA." It's worth every penny and we strongly recommend it.

In summary, make sure you get all the pain relief and medication you need. Tell the physicians and nurses if the pain medicine you're getting is not adequate. Demerol, Morphine, Nubain or Toradol will often be the first injectable agent given. Any of these is fine, but if the first medicine doesn't work, it might be a good idea to ask for an adjustment in the dosage or suggest they try a combination. If you are nauseous, be sure to ask for an anti-nausea medication along with the pain relievers. And if you're admitted to the hospital for pain control, but sure to ask for "PCA."

CHAPTER FOUR

Your Visit to the Emergency Room

For many of you reading this book, your first visit to the Emergency Room (ER) may have been caused by a kidney stone. It was probably a memorable experience! The ER is actually the best place to be with an acute pain attack from a stone. The ER staff are prepared to rapidly check laboratory values from blood and urine samples, obtain X-rays or other imaging studies, make a quick but accurate diagnosis, and monitor your condition while giving you intravenous fluid, as well as the pain medicine you desperately need to get through the stone attack. They will contact your doctor or assign one to you if you don't have one. Knowing how an Emergency Room really works will make your visit less frightening, as well as improve your medical care and subsequent treatment.

If you've watched the television show "ER," you may have noticed that they rarely have shown any patients with kidney stones. It's probably because stones are not "flashy" like gun shots or accidents. Don't expect a real emergency room to be like the one on television!

When to Go to the Emergency Room

If you have a sudden, severe pain attack in the side or back which radiates to the groin area and is accompanied by nausea or vomiting, then there is a good chance that you have a kidney stone. If you don't have a stone, then there's something serious going on anyway and you should still go to the nearest hospital Emergency Room.

Doctors recommend a hospital ER because they are staffed 24 hours a day with specially trained personnel who have access to all the necessary technology to make a diagnosis and can prescribe painkillers and antibiotics as necessary. (Other procedures may need to be performed that urgent care centers and many doctor's offices are not able to do).

Depending on your medical insurance plan, you may need to contact your regular doctor to guarantee coverage. Be aware that unless he or she is an expert in stone disease and has a full laboratory and X-ray facilities in the office, you may not have access to the full range of services you need.

Try not to urinate before you go to the ER because they will almost certainly ask you for a urine sample to check for traces of blood, crystals and infection. Bring a list of any medicines you may be taking. Be prepared to stay in the hospital if it becomes necessary, and don't eat or drink anything once you've made the decision to go to the ER.

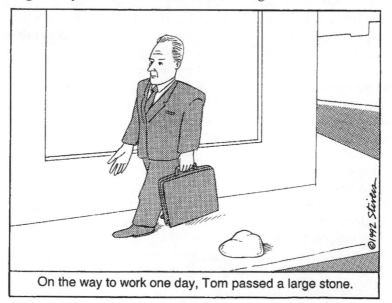

On the way to work one day, Tom passed a large stone.

Reprinted with permission; Mark Stivers, Sacramento, CA.

Don't Drive Yourself to the Emergency Room!

If you are in so much pain that you can't think straight, you shouldn't drive either! Have a friend or relative take you. If no one is available, call a taxi or an ambulance, but never drive if you think you may have a kidney stone. A car accident will not improve your chances of getting the stone treated!

When you get to the hospital, make sure you tell them what's wrong. The staff will not be aware of all your symptoms and problems just by looking at you (although they can make a good guess at most stone patients just by the way we moan and groan). If you've had a previous stone and this feels "just like the last stone attack," it's OK to tell them, but don't be overbearing. You would be surprised how often it turns out to be something else like diverticulitis (an infection of the large intestine) or appendicitis. Let the ER doctors do whatever testing they feel is necessary. That's what they are trained to do. After all, you wouldn't want them to make a mistake!

How A Kidney Stone is Diagnosed

Usually, the diagnosis is fairly obvious. Typically, patients are in severe pain which started suddenly. They clutch their back or sides and move constantly, unable to find any comfortable position. (By contrast, someone with an acute appendicitis will usually want to stay absolutely motionless). ER personnel will check your urine for blood, crystals and infection. While not everyone with a stone will show microscopic blood in the urine, over 85 percent do, and its presence helps make the diagnosis easier.

Some type of imaging study is usually done next. A flat plate of the abdomen or KUB (Kidney, Ureter and Bladder) film will probably be taken. Other imaging studies will then be selected by the ER physician based on the individual situation.

Until recently, the standard diagnostic X-ray was the Intravenous Pyelogram (IVP), or kidney X-rays. Special contrast or dye is given to the patient through a needle into a vein. The contrast is filtered from the blood by the kidneys, allowing them to show up clearly on X-ray. Without the dye, the kidneys would be almost invisible to standard X-rays. If there is a long delay for the contrast to filter into one of the kidneys, this is very suggestive of a stone causing a sudden blockage.

After the procedure, you may be asked to wait until all the dye has filtered through the kidneys; this can take many hours if there is a blockage. There is also the slight danger of an allergic reaction to the dye itself. Make sure you ask for the "non-ionic" dye, which is less likely to cause an allergic reaction.

Another form of imaging study being done quite often in many ERs for kidney stones is the CT (Computerized Tomography) scan. The CT scanner is a very large machine that looks something like a doughnut where the patient is placed in the "hole." An X-ray machine is built into the wall of the doughnut where is circles the patient's body, taking a number of small X-rays. A special computer then creates pictures based on these little X-rays.

The advantages of the CT scan are that it is relatively quick and requires no contrast medium, it shows stones that are not easily seen on the IVP, and it can often help make a diagnosis even if the problem doesn't happen to be a kidney stone. The disadvantage is that the CT scan is often a bit more expensive than the IVP and may not give sufficient detail for the urologist to plan a surgical procedure or approach. Rarely, stones are invisible even to the CT scanner. These usually occur in patients taking certain medications called Protease Inhibitors. Be sure to tell the ER doctors if you are taking any protease inhibitor medications.

(Dr. Leslie's personal preference is to go with the CT scan if it's available to get a quick diagnosis. He feels an IVP can be performed later if necessary).

Not every CT scanner is suitable for a kidney stone study. The scanner must have sufficient resolution and take views, or "slices,"very close together, usually no more than 1/2 cm. (or about 1/4 inch) apart, for the study to be considered reliable. The ER physicians will know if the type of CT scanner they have available is the right kind to do a kidney stone or "renal colic" study (renal colic is the medical term doctors use for the severe pain cause by a sudden kidney stone attack).

Don't be afraid to talk to the nurses and doctors in the ER. If the type of medication they give you isn't working or the dosage is not adequate after a reasonable period of time, don't be afraid to tell someone. If you're experiencing nausea, a doctor can give you some medication to relieve it. If they advise you to stay in the hospital, it's usually a good idea to heed their advice. The way things are now in medicine, a patient is almost never urged to stay in the hospital without a very good reason. Ask the doctor to explain the reason.

How to Find Good Kidney Stone Doctor

Once they have established that you have a stone, the ER staff will either contact your regular doctor or assign you to one on call. Your regular doctor may refer you to a urology specialist. If so, make sure the urologist is qualified as noted below. You may not have a choice about the physician assigned to you in the ER since this is based on a rotating schedule of the doctors on staff.

Ask for a urologist if possible, because urologists are the specialists who are most knowledgeable about kidney stones and will ultimately have to decide whether some type of surgery is necessary. Ask the nurses and ER physicians if there is a urologist or other medical expert in the community who has a special interest or skill in kidney stone prevention. This is the specialist you will eventually want to contact. But that may have to wait until the immediate stone problem is resolved. You can also call the National Kidney Stone Patient Network at 1-800- 2KIDNEYS where a database of kidney stone prevention specialists is maintained.

One technique is to ask the ER personnel who "they " would see for kidney stones. Make sure the urologist is Board Certified. This means he or she has taken all the required years of training and passed a series of rigorous examinations. Although many excellent urologists are not Board Certified, if you have a choice why not pick one who is? This can be checked on the Internet or through the American Urological Association (AUA) who will give you a list of the Board Certified urologists in your community. The AUA can be contacted at (410) 727-1100.

Staying in the Hospital

There are several good reasons why you should stay in the hospital following a kidney stone attack:

- unrelenting pain which requires medication either through an IV or by injection.

- severe nausea and vomiting which would lead to dehydration and prevent you from taking oral pain medication.

- infection or fever which could lead to serious bacterial blood poisoning (sepsis).

- if you have only one working kidney which is now blocked with a stone.

- kidney failure or some other serious medical disorder.

For many patients, one or two shots of painkiller may provide enough relief to allow them to go home. This is because the painkiller causes the spasms to decrease as the system slowly adjusts to the blockage and urine begins to pass around the stone, limiting any further stretching or dilating. When this happens, the stone pain and discomfort disappear. Of course, you could also pass the stone completely out of your body—which is why you'll be asked to strain all your urine. It's very important to catch any stone fragments for later analysis.

"Admission" Versus "Observation"

Once upon a time, the decision to admit a patient to a hospital was simply up to the discretion of the physician after a discussion with the patient. In the current world of managed care, this often becomes a wrestling match between you, your doctor, and the insurance company. It is now very rare to be formally admitted to a hospital with a stone. Rather, you are "observed." You still stay in the hospital in a room and bed, but it's still considered "observation" unless you need to stay more than 24 hours. The reason is that most patients are able to go home within this time, and the insurance companies often insist on this "word game." It shouldn't make any difference to you as long as you receive the care you need and aren't shuffled out the door before you're ready.

The criteria for discharge from the hospital are the same as for the ER:

- The pain needs to be controlled adequately with medication you can safely take at home.

- You need to be able to eat or at least drink sufficient amounts of fluids.

- You do not have a fever or signs of infection.

If you are asked to go home before you are ready, object!

Make sure you ask for a strainer to check for any stones in your urine and for a prescription for pain medication and/or an antibiotic.

Straining the Urine

Paint strainers and aquarium nets generally make the best urinary stone strainers. In Dr. Leslie's office, an aquarium net, available in most pet stores, is recommended because it's durable, reusable, comes in multiple sizes, has a nice wire handle to keep one's hands clean and possesses a fine, tight, white nylon mesh in which even the smallest stones can easily be seen. It is reusable after washing. The strainer should be carried with you at all times and used every single time your urinate until the stone is collected or your physician tells you to stop.

Portable, small-sized strainers are also available upon request by writing to Four Geez Press. These small strainers can slip into a coat pocket or purse and allow you to return to your normal activities without announcing to the world you're collecting kidney stones.

Ask for Your X-Rays

When you arrive for the appointment following an emergency room visit, make sure you bring any stone fragments you passed and all of the X-rays that were taken while you were in the hospital. In some cases, the hospital will not release the X- rays until they are officially reviewed or "read" by a radiologist (a physician who specializes in the interpretation of X-rays and other imaging studies). This usually takes about one business day. After that, most hospitals will allow you to take your films to your doctor's office for further review, or ask them to make copies for you.

CHAPTER FIVE

Diagnosing Kidney Stones

How do you know you *really* have a kidney stone?

A preliminary diagnosis can be made from your medical history and a physical examination. You may have had an attack which began with severe pain in the upper side and back. The pain may have radiated down the side towards the lower abdomen and finally groin. Nausea and vomiting may have added to your discomfort. Adding further misery, you may have also experienced urinary frequency, urgency and possibly bladder spasms.

A physical examination can sometimes be difficult because patients with kidney stone pain (colic) tend to be constantly moving, trying to find a comfortable position. Most patients with serious bowel problems, an acute abdomen or appendicitis will try to lie absolutely still. A light tapping of the upper back over the kidney may cause severe and intense pain. Fever is uncommon unless there is a urinary infection. If a fever is present, then the stone attack becomes a potentially more serious problem and antibiotics will be needed.

A urine examination, called a urinalysis, will be necessary. The urine will usually show at least some microscopic blood. It will also be examined for the presence of any bacteria or infection. While blood in the urine is a classic sign for kidney stones, about 10 to 15 percent of patients with known stones may not have any visible or microscopic blood in their urine!

Imaging

Every patient with a possible kidney stone requires some type of imaging study of the urinary tract. The most common forms of imaging are ultrasound, intravenous pyelogram (IVP), retrograde pyelograms and computerized tomography (CT) scans. Other studies, such as a single flat X-ray of the abdomen (called a "KUB" for kidneys, ureters and bladder), and especially plain tomograms of the kidneys are useful in following the progress of stone disease. Each of these studies is reviewed in detail below.

Ultrasound

Ultrasound is the name of an imaging machine that uses high frequency sound waves to look into the body and make pictures. These sound waves cannot be heard and are totally painless and harmless to the body. The sound waves bounce off body structures, stones and organs. The echoes are picked up by a microphone and the signals processed into a black and white picture.

The image looks a little like snow at night with a very dark background and lots of little white dots. However, to an expert, the pattern of these white dots indicates the anatomy and internal structure of the area being scanned. Ultrasound is similar to the sonar used in submarines to identify nearby objects.

In practice, ultrasound is quick, cheap, safe and painless. While it may not always show the stone, it is reasonably good at finding the stretching or dilating of the upper urinary system and kidney caused by a blockage of the ureter.

The dilation of the kidney and upper ureter is called hydronephrosis and it usually means that some type of obstruction is present downstream even though the location of such a blockage may not be seen.

Unfortunately, ultrasound is not very clear or precise and it cannot reliably identify most stones, especially if they are small and outside the kidney.

Intravenous Pyelogram (IVP)

The Intravenous Pyelogram or IVP has been the gold standard for the diagnosis of kidney stones for many years. It is being replaced in many institutions by CT scans which are faster, safer and more likely to help make a diagnosis if a stone is not present.

An IVP is a series of X-rays performed immediately after administration of a special contrast agent or dye directly into a vein. An intravenous fluid line is started and a simple X-ray is done before the contrast is given. After the dye has been injected, additional X-rays are taken. The contrast flows through the blood or vascular system and eventually is excreted by the kidneys. This contrast makes the kidney tissue appear somewhat gray and the urine white. Without contrast, the urinary system and kidneys are totally dark and almost impossible to see.

If there is a stone blocking a ureter, the kidney on that side will take much longer to excrete the contrast. During this time, the affected kidney will fill up with contrast and appear much whiter than the unaffected kidney. This is called the "nephrogram effect" and it is an important clue that there is a stone or at least an obstruction on that side. While a normal IVP may take only 30 to 40 minutes to complete, with a severe obstruction from a stone it can take many hours for the contrast to slowly work its way down the ureter to the point of obstruction. These later X-rays pictures, called delay films, are essential to precisely identify the location of the stone.

IVP's are excellent for making a diagnosis of kidney stones. Calcium stones will show up clearly and their exact location can be pinpointed. Non-calcium stones can be much harder to see, but their effect on slowing the passage of the contrast and stretching of the urinary system upstream from the obstruction is usually sufficient for a diagnosis.

There are problems associated with IVP's. The time needed to obtain a complete set of films, which can take many hours in some cases, can be excessive. Patients with diabetes or kidney failure may suffer some kidney damage from the contrast. X-rays in pregnant women need to be minimized. An intravenous line needs to be started. Some patients will be allergic to the contrast or dye.

Patients with mild or moderate allergies can be pretreated with antihistamines and a brief course of steroids over several days and proceed safely with the IVP, but patients with severe allergies to intravenous contrast should probably not have any intravenous contrast at all. Fortunately, there are other means to evaluate stones that do not require exposure to intravenous contrast.

Retrograde Pyelograms

Retrograde pyelograms can be used to examine the urinary system including the ureters and inside of the kidneys even in patients with severe allergies to contrast media. Retrograde refers to the direction of the contrast which is injected into the lower, downstream end of the ureter and allowed to pass upwards through the ureter and into the kidney. Pyelogram refers to a picture of the internal urine collection sack of the kidney called the renal pelvis.

First, a cystoscopy or visual telescopic inspection of the bladder must be done. Under anesthesia, a small specially designed telescope is gently passed into the bladder through the urethra or penis. The telescope allows the operator to find the tiny opening of the ureter into the bladder. A small, thin tube is then directed into this opening and the contrast is injected. A quick X-ray film is taken when the entire urinary system is filled with the dye. Any blockage, stone, narrowing or kinking will be apparent on the film. Usually this technique gives a very clear picture, even more precise than the IVP and there is no risk of any allergic response since the contrast never reaches the bloodstream. Still, it is somewhat difficult and tedious to perform, it requires anesthesia and there is the possibility it could introduce bacteria and infection into the urinary system. Usually, other imaging techniques are preferred whenever possible.

CT (Computerized Tomography) Scans

CT scans use a large, round machine and a computer to create a series of images or pictures of the human body. These scans are usually performed with IV (intravenous), oral and sometimes rectal contrast used to help identify the intestines, bowel and urinary system. This is the same contrast used in the IVP. Each scan from the machine creates a computerized image of the patient at the level of the scan.

Recently, CT scans using the newest generation of scanners and without any contrast have been used for diagnosis in patients suspected of having kidney stone attacks. Each scan is positioned so close to the previous scan that there is very little chance that even a small stone will escape detection. Without contrast to mask the appearance of any stones, they are usually easy to see. If the patient has some other medical problem instead of a kidney stone, such as a ruptured appendix, bowel obstruction or abdominal aneurysm, there is a good chance that this will be correctly identified on the CT scan. The scan can be done quickly and there is no risk of allergic reactions if no contrast is used. The only drawback is that the machine is more expensive to operate than a standard X-ray machine so the cost may be higher in some institutions. While additional X-rays may be needed if surgery or ESWL is necessary, the CT scan is rapidly becoming the diagnostic imaging technique of choice for patients who come to the emergency room with a possible kidney stone attack. It is particularly useful in older patients where other medical problems can easily be confused with kidney stones.

Flat Plate or KUB (Kidneys, Ureters and Bladder)

A plain film or flat plate of the abdomen and pelvis, often called a KUB for Kidneys, Ureters and Bladder, is often the first imaging technique used in a case of suspected kidney stones. Most stones contain calcium and will show up on these X- rays. Unfortunately, many people who have multiple small, round calcified spots on their X-rays in areas that could possibly indicate stones. These calcium containing spots are usually phleboliths. Phleboliths are calcifications that naturally occur in the veins particularly where there are small valves. They would not be important clinically except that they can look a little like calcium kidney stones. It may take an IVP, CT scan or Retrograde Pyelogram to tell the difference.

The KUB is fast and often helpful, but it may not be adequate for a correct diagnosis. It is probably most helpful in monitoring the progress of a stone already identified by other means. It is also used to check on the passage of the stone particles after fragmentation by the ESWL machine.

Plain Renal Tomograms

It can often be difficult or impossible to identify some stone located inside the kidney due to overlying bowel contents or gas. Plain, meaning non-contrast, tomograms are X-rays made with a rotating machine that is able to focus at various levels within the kidney. (Renal just means pertaining to the kidney.) Only those structures located at the focus levels of the X-ray will be visible and everything else will disappear. The photographic plate and the X-ray source both rotate around the patient in opposite directions. The center of rotation, located at some point inside the patient, becomes the focal point of the X-ray. Nothing actually touches the patient and there are no needles, incisions or pain. The techniques gives very clear pictures and even small stones can be seen clearly, but it takes several films to scan the entire kidney and a special X-ray machine to do the studies. Plain renal tomograms are often underutilized by many medical professionals.

With one or more of these imaging techniques, it should be possible to correctly identify any and all stones that might be present in the urinary system.

CHAPTER SIX

Suggestions and Tips for Selecting Realistic Preventive Treatment

Did you know that jade got its name because the Spanish conquistadors of Mexico thought the green stones carved by the native people could cure kidney complaints? They called them "kidney stones"or "piedras de ijada" (literally stone of the flank). If only curing kidney stone woes were as simple as buying some jade jewelry!

The preventive medical management of a kidney stone patient can be challenging even to an experienced specialist. Many patients ask, "What can I expect from a good prevention plan?"

Let's get serious. Preventing kidney stones requires hard work and a lifetime commitment to achieving good health. Patients who have endured the pain and frustration of even a single kidney stone are willing to follow the basics of any reasonable stone prevention plan.

Once 24-hour metabolic urine testing is completed, dietary modifications are encouraged to eliminate any obvious excesses which can result in further stone growth. One example is to reduce excessive consumption of meat and meat by-products especially in patients who form uric acid stones (excess protein is converted to uric acid).

Secondly, drinking enough fluids sufficient to maintain a daily urinary volume of 2000 cc's or more (roughly a half gallon) is important. Adequate fluid intake is a universally accepted fact in stone prevention. If these measures fail to reduce the high risk factors, then medication will be needed.

When formulating a treatment plan, you and your physician should start with a 24-hour urine metabolic stone risk test. You should consider the following:

- Dependability and completeness of the laboratory studies. Many clinical and hospital laboratories perform urine chemistry testing infrequently or with inadequate quality controls. Be certain that the laboratory conducting your urine chemistry testing performs these particular analyses often, has a good reputation for reliability and rigorous quality standards. We recommend any of the commercial labs listed in Chapter Ten that specialize in this particular testing.

- Your willingness to follow specific treatment options. If you're not reasonably willing to adhere to specific treatment recommendations for an indefinite period, then the likelihood of long-term success is reduced. Please tell the doctor if you are unable or unwilling to follow any particular therapy.

- If multiple chemical problems are detected, treat the most significant or potentially dangerous ones first and select the simplest possible therapy.

- Likelihood of long-term patient compliance and follow-up testing. Certain treatments are more likely than others to be followed regularly by the majority of patients. A difficult treatment or one with significant side effects is unlikely to be tolerated by most people over months and years of therapy.

- Probability of side effects and complications. Communicate any problems with your urologist. Dialogue is important. For example, one prescription drug (Urocit-K) is eliminated from the body as an intact tablet apparently unchanged after passing through the digestive tract. This is completely normal for this particular medication. Some patients misjudge this and think they are not absorbing the drug. Physicians need to alert patients to this possibility.

■ Treatment effectiveness and safety. Whenever possible, only the safest and most effective therapies should be used. For example, overly aggressive reduction in calcium intake should be avoided. Severe dietary calcium restrictions may liberate other minerals in the intestinal tract which normally bind with calcium, such as oxalate, resulting in an increase in absorption of these stone promoting chemicals. A dietary calcium restriction of less than 400 mg. per day is not recommended and usually 600 to 800 mg. is sufficient. This is roughly equivalent to one good calcium or dairy meal per day. Also, lowering salt intake is beneficial since salt in the urine is associated with a high urinary calcium excretion.

Patients with calcium oxalate stones who have elevated urinary uric acid levels (hyperuricosuria) will usually normalize the uric acid with dietary moderation from a high protein intake. Severe protein restriction is not required or advisable. Patients who form pure uric acid stones usually do not respond to dietary protein restriction alone and will require allopurinol and citrate therapy, both prescription medications.

■ Routine follow-up testing is essential to determine the effectiveness of therapy and to identify any new high risk factors which might appear. Physicians have found this happens surprisingly often. This is frequently due to dietary adjustments. When restrictions are placed on one particular food item, most patients will increase consumption of a substitute which may have new and unpredictable effects on stone production.

■ Remember that the "best" therapy on paper may be unacceptable to you as the patient or ineffective when implemented. Careful discussion with your doctor together with routine follow-up testing will help in optimizing treatment.

■ A complete X-ray survey of any existing stones should be done before starting therapy. This can usually be accomplished with an IVP or plain renal tomograms. This is necessary so the physician can determine whether any additional stones that are passed existed prior to starting therapy.

■ It is often difficult for some patients to achieve the optimal level of urine production of 2000 cc's or more per day. Many patients will rebel or just simply fail to improve if merely told to go home and drink 8 glasses of water a day. Increasing fluid intake significantly is not easy, but if you follow any increased fluid intake regimen for just a few months, your body's fluid thermostat will reset and you will get thirsty if your fluid consumption level should drop.

Thiazides, a class of water pill or diuretic, can be used as a last resort to increase urinary volume. Thiazides will force an obligatory increase in urinary volume—but there is a risk of becoming dehydrated if your fluid intake doesn't increase accordingly. Thiazides are also used to treat high urinary calcium. They remove calcium from the urine and return it to the bloodstream. When using thiazides to treat high urinary calcium levels, be aware of its potential side effects on other chemicals. Thiazides can decrease potassium in the blood, increase uric acid and decrease urine citrate levels. Anticipating these difficulties, we recommend that thiazides be used together with potassium citrate supplements in the majority of cases, even if the urinary citrate is not initially decreased. Thiazides may eventually lose their urinary calcium lowering effect. Therefore, periodic rechecks are essential.

An increase in urinary oxalate is chemically a much greater contributor to new stone formation than a proportionate increase in urinary calcium. Sometimes increasing dietary calcium can reduce calcium oxalate stone production. Consider magnesium or iron dietary supplements as substitute intestinal oxalate binding agents.

Other Factors Which Lower Stone Risk

When no specific high risk factor is obvious, it may be beneficial to concentrate on other factors which lower stone risk. Make sure you do not make any major changes in lifestyle, diet or medications prior to or during testing. It may be useful to repeat the entire testing protocol in several months if stone growth or production continues.

Many physicians recommend trying dietary therapies first. Usually only moderate adjustments are necessary. We rarely exclude any food entirely. If you do "cheat" and eat a dietary product on the "restricted" list, you must pay a "penalty" and drink at least two extra glasses of water to help dilute the effect.

Now that we have outlined the essentials, in the following chapters we'll guide you through these medical stone prevention techniques and therapies in greater detail.

CHAPTER SEVEN

Uric Acid Stones
"The Invisible Menace"

P rior to discussing uric acid, this is a good time to explain another quirky habit about kidney stones. Even in the same family, brothers or sisters can make different kidney stones. My brother is a master at creating uric acid stones. Mine tend to be the more common calcium oxalate variety. The pain is still the same, however, so our combined goal is to prevent all "homemade" kidney stones.

Men are more likely than women to get uric acid problems which may result in gout, uric acid stones, calcium oxalate stones or all three. Uric acid stones account for about five to ten percent of the total incidence of renal stones.

Uric acid is a primarily a waste product from the breakdown of purine. Purine is one of the chemical building blocks of the genetic code material (DNA and RNA) found inside every living cell. Purines in the body normally come from three sources:

■ Genetic material from cells that are being routinely destroyed by the body because of damage or age. This is a continuous, normal process that allows the body to replace old or damaged cells with new ones.

■ Production of new purine molecules by the body to form the genetic code material for any new cells being formed.

■ Digestion of purines from the diet. This normally accounts for less than half of the uric acid produced, but it's usually responsible for most of the problems from increased uric acid levels. Protein rich foods that are high in purines include red meat, pork, poultry and fish. Other high purine foods include grapes, instant coffee, berries, citrus fruits, juices, and certain vegetables. Still more foods to avoid include alcohol, sardines, anchovies, herring and organ meats such as liver.

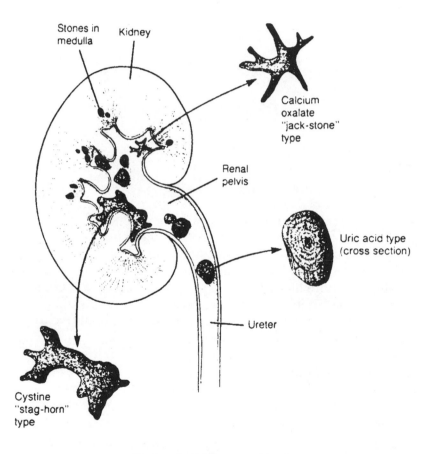

Stones in kidney and ureter.

Reprinted with permission from Times Mirror Mosby College Publishing, *Nutrition & Diet Therapy* by Sue Rodwell Williams, Ph.D., M.P.H., R.D., 5th Edition, 1985.

Too much uric acid in the urine is called hyperuricosuria. This can result from eating an excessive amount of meat, fish or poultry and is often controlled if the patient changes their diet.

Patients who have had a part of their large intestine removed will lose extra antacid (citrate and bicarbonate) which is normally absorbed by that organ. Their bodies will tend to become more acidic and excrete less antacid (citrate) in the urine. They also tend to become dehydrated due to water loss and thus are prone to uric acid stone formation.

The liver chemically treats excess purine until it finally forms uric acid. Some uric acid is eliminated through the digestive tract where it is broken down by intestinal bacteria. Most of the body's uric acid, about two thirds, is eventually filtered from the blood by the kidneys and excreted in the urine.

The bad news is that uric acid doesn't dissolve very easily in either water or urine. The higher the acid content, the less uric acid can dissolve. Most animals continue the chemical conversion of uric acid a few more critical steps and create allantoin which is up to 100 times easier to dissolve than uric acid. Only Dalmatian dogs, higher apes and humans have lost the ability to make allantoin from uric acid and we therefore share a problem of uric acid excretion and stone formation. Human uric acid levels are generally 10 times greater than most other animals. Patients with high uric acid levels in either their blood or urine are at increased risk to make both uric acid and calcium oxalate stones.

A number of medications can affect uric acid production or excretion. Aspirin and similar compounds, probenicid, steroids, various cancer chemotherapy agents, alcohol, thiazides and lasix are all known to increase uric acid levels in either the blood, urine or both.

Allopurinol

Allopurinol is a medication that stops the formation of uric acid through a chemical block. Another chemical called Xanthine then becomes the end product of protein digestion instead of uric acid. Xanthine will dissolve in urine much easier than uric acid and rarely forms stones. Allopurinol is used primarily in cases of gout and in pure uric acid stones. (More details about allopurinol will be found in the next chapter on calcium).

Urinary Antacids

Urinary antacids, also called alkalinizing agents, are those medicines or supplements which will reduce acid levels in the body and urine. Urinary antacid therapy is the treatment of choice for kidney stone patients with renal tubular acidosis, cystine stones or low urinary citrate and are particularly useful in the chemical dissolution and prevention of uric acid stones.

Neutralizing excess urinary acid can be accomplished in several ways when dietary methods alone are insufficient. The most useful antacid agents are oral supplements of sodium bicarbonate and potassium citrate. Both will increase urinary citrate (antacid) levels. Oral antacids containing potassium are usually preferred because the extra potassium tends to lower urinary calcium excretion while sodium increases it. Potassium citrate has the advantage of both liquid and tablet availability, simultaneous potassium supplementation and a more uniform effect. Depending on the antacid, the patient will need to monitor their urinary acid level to keep it within the desired parameters.

Urinary antacid therapy should not be used in infection (struvite) stone formers and only cautiously in patients with calcium phosphate stones since calcium phosphate tends to form more readily as urinary acid levels drop. One important example is renal tubular acidosis, a condition where the kidney is unable to excrete excess acid into the urine. Renal tubular acidosis is characterized by calcium phosphate stones, high blood acid levels, low urinary citrate excretion and a persistently low urinary acid. Oral antacid therapy is required and potassium citrate is usually the preferred treatment.

Gout and "Gouty Diathesis"

Gout is the condition where blood levels of uric acid are consistently elevated. It can cause uric acid crystals to form inside joints and create a type of painful arthritis. Treatment for gout is usually allopurinol, a medication that blocks the formation of uric acid, or one of several anti-inflammatory medications which treat the arthritis. In some cases, patients will be placed on medications that increase uric acid excretion in the urine. This reduces the blood uric acid level and lowers the risk of a gout attack, but it obviously increases the chances for uric acid kidney stones. Aspirin, probenicid and thiazides are examples of such medications.

About 25 percent of all patients with gout will eventually form urinary stones. Many gout patients will excrete normal amounts of urinary uric acid, but will demonstrate instead a very acid urine. This extremely acid urine will promote both uric acid and calcium oxalate kidney stone formation. This condition, where gout is associated with kidney stone formation, is called "Gouty Diathesis." It is usually treated with potassium citrate supplements to neutralize the extremely acid urine. If high urinary uric acid levels are present, then allopurinol may be added. Dietary protein restrictions are generally not practical or effective in this condition, but excessively high meat protein intake should still be discouraged.

Uric Acid Stones

Pure uric acid stones are not generally visible on standard X-rays, although they can usually be seen on CT scans. A standard kidney X-ray (called an intravenous pyelogram or IVP) may not show the actual stone, but it will demonstrate the level of blockage and the absence of any visible calcium. A diagnosis of uric acid stones is more likely if the blood uric acid level is increased (a condition called gout) or if the urine has a high acid level with a pH of 5.5 or less. Dehydration and chronic diarrhea can increase uric acid stone production.

Pure uric acid stones account for between 5 percent and 10 percent of all urinary stones and will occur in about 1 out of every 1,000 people in the United States. By contrast, 75 percent of all kidney stones in Israel are composed of uric acid. The most important factors in uric acid stone production are:

1. High Urinary Uric Acid Levels
2. High Urinary Acidity
3. Relatively Low Urinary Volumes
4. High Serum Uric Acid
5. Excessive Dietary Protein Intake

Treatment of Uric Acid Stones

Uric acid dissolves best in an antacid (scientifically, this is also called alkaline or basic) solution. It's therefore possible to dissolve uric acid stones if we can reduce the acid content of the urine sufficiently. This can be done by IV administration of antacids in a hospital. Sometimes it's possible to irrigate or rinse uric acid stones with an antacid solution and dissolve them. Typically, many physicians use oral potassium citrate supplementation. Sufficient oral citrate to maintain the urine pH between 6.5 and 7.0. is usually recommended. (Urinary acid is normally measured by pH where 7.0 is considered "neutral" like plain water. The lower the pH number, the greater the amount of acidity.) In most cases, allopurinol therapy is begun to reduce the amount of uric acid being produced and excreted into the urine. Allopurinol also makes it easier to regulate the urinary pH within optimal levels by reducing overall urinary acid excretion.

The urinary pH can be easily measured by use of special pH paper which turns a characteristic color at each pH level. The amount of potassium citrate supplementation can then be adjusted as necessary to maintain an optimal urinary acid level. If chemically dissolving the stones doesn't work, then standard surgical stone treatments will be needed.

What is pH and Why Is It Important?

pH is a measurement of the acid level of any liquid. If the pH is high, then the liquid has very little acid compared to water and is called alkaline or basic. If the pH is low, the liquid contains more acid than water and is called acidic. (Water is considered "neutral" and is arbitrarily given a pH value of 7.0). Urine normally is slightly acid with a pH usually between 5 and 7. A specially treated paper than turns a specific color for each pH level is currently available but it can be hard to read since it was not originally designed for testing urine acid levels. A special disposable dipstick should be ready for purchase soon which will make it easier for patients to monitor the pH levels and various other chemical properties of the urine when instructed to do so (see the Resource Section at the back of the book for more information about this new dipstick for stone formers).

Particularly for pure uric acid stones, monitoring the pH is vital in preventing more stones from forming. This requires taking special urinary antacid supplements of either sodium bicarbonate or potassium citrate periodically. (Urologists prefer potassium citrate for the reasons reviewed earlier). Too little antacid means that the urine will remain very acid and the uric acid won't dissolve. Too much antacid and another stone forming compound, calcium phosphate, can begin to form which creates new problems. For uric acid stones, the goal is generally to keep the urinary pH roughly between 6.5 and 7. Ten times more uric acid can dissolve at a pH of 7.0 than at a pH of 5.5. If the pH is too low, indicating too much acid, the patient should increase his supplemental potassium citrate therapy. If the pH is too high, the patient should reduce the potassium citrate intake.

J. Smith was 65 years-old when he first came to see Dr. Leslie. He had heard about Dr. Leslie's stone prevention program in the local newspaper and made the appointment almost as a last resort. He claimed to have passed over 50 separate stones over the previous five years. That would mean about one per month! While this is certainly a large number of stones, it isn't a world's record. Some patients seen in Dr. Leslie's office have made 500 stones. Mr. Smith had undergone two separate open surgeries for kidney stone disease and had been under the care of three other physicians before being seen by Dr. Leslie. Only one kidney was functioning and it had several stones in it.

None of his stones had ever been analyzed. He brought some from home and Dr. Leslie had them analyzed. They were pure uric acid. He was started on allopurinol and citrate supplements. He dissolved his remaining stones and has stayed stone free ever since. His metabolic analysis showed that he had normal amounts of uric acid, calcium and oxalate but had a very acid urine. He asked Dr. Leslie several years later why none of the other doctors he'd seen had bothered to analyze the stones, offer preventive testing or prescribe the same medicine? It might have been just overlooked. Regardless, it was clearly a mistake not to pursue metabolic testing and treatment in this individual.

Long-term treatment and prevention of uric acid stones usually requires allopurinol and often some regular citrate supplementation which helps by neutralizing excess urinary acid. This can often be done only once a day at bedtime. Normally, the urine produced during the night has less acid than during the day. This event may be the body's way of helping to prevent uric acid crystals and stones from developing. When citrate is taken before bed, it will enhance and strengthen this normal nighttime process.

In children, certain medical disorders such as acute leuke-mia can cause very significant elevations in uric acid. This would primarily occur during chemotherapy as a result of the death and destruction of the cancer being treated. As the cancer cells die, they produce a large purine load for the body to chemically break down which ultimately results in a uric acid excess. Patients at risk are often placed on allopurinol prior to any chemotherapy for this reason.

Review Capsule: As a general rule, pure uric acid stones are treated with allopurinol while calcium ox-alate stones formed in elevated urinary uric acid con-ditions are treated first with citrate and dietary mod-eration of red meat, poultry and fish. Many cases will require all of these remedies. Increased fluid intake is also essential.

CHAPTER EIGHT

Bones, Stones, Moans and Groans: Calcium and Stone Disease

Excessive urinary calcium is the one most common metabolic risk factor for kidney stone disease. There are many causes but the most common is increased intestinal calcium absorption.

When other causes, such Renal Phosphate Leak, Hyperparathyroidism and Hypervitaminosis D (all reviewed later in this chapter) have been eliminated by blood tests, the only remaining diagnoses are increased intestinal calcium absorption and renal calcium leak. The test which distinguishes between them is called a Calcium Loading Test. There are usually enough clues to suggest either increased intestinal calcium absorption or renal calcium leak as the cause of any abnormally high levels of urinary calcium without having to do the Calcium Loading Test.

First, the patient is placed on a very strict low calcium, low salt diet to follow for one week. Urine samples for calcium are taken before and after a large prepared calcium supplement "meal." If urinary calcium returns to normal on the strict low calcium diet, but increases significantly after the high calcium meal, then increased intestinal calcium absorption is present. If there is little difference between the two readings or if the urinary calcium on the strict low calcium diet remains elevated, then there are two possibilities: either the kidneys are unable to retain calcium in the bloodstream so calcium "leaks" into the urine in high amounts (thus, called renal calcium leak) or a hormonal problem is present.

Fortunately, a simple blood test for calcium and hormone levels will easily determine which is present.

The Calcium Loading Test is difficult to perform and interpret. For most patients, standard 24 hour urine tests and a brief trial of therapy should give the same conclusion without the need for this complicated test.

A simple, moderately low calcium diet trial is often enough to demonstrate the effectiveness of dietary therapy alone in reducing urinary calcium excretion. Urinary calcium that returns to normal using only a moderately low calcium diet should be treated with dietary therapy. If dietary measures alone are unsuccessful, then medical therapy with thiazides, orthophosphates, allopurinol, potassium citrate and possibly cellulose and magnesium will be needed.

Increased Intestinal Calcium Absorption (Absorptive Hypercalciuria)

Patients with increased intestinal calcium absorption (absorptive hypercalciuria) tend to have normal or slightly low levels of serum parathyroid hormone while those with renal calcium leak usually have relatively large amounts of this hormone in the blood (parathyroid hormone increases the blood calcium level). Increased intestinal calcium absorption is by far the most common known cause of high urinary calcium levels. Patients are advised not to try to limit their dietary intake of calcium beyond a moderate, reasonable amount. Recent studies have shown that too drastic a restriction on dietary calcium will actually increase stone recurrence rates. This will be explained in Chapter Nine.

There are two clinical varieties of increased intestinal calcium absorption:

■ Type I: Unresponsive to a moderately low calcium diet but controllable with the addition of cellulose therapy (cellulose is a very strong binder of calcium in the diet) or:

■ Type II: Responsive to a moderately low calcium diet alone.

Patients who are unresponsive to both a reasonably low calcium diet and cellulose probably don't have increased intestinal calcium absorption.

What is Renal Calcium Leak?

Renal calcium leak is a condition where the kidneys release a large amount of calcium into the urine regardless of the blood calcium level. These patients will show a high obligatory loss of blood calcium into the urine even when the blood calcium level is low! Patients do not respond well to low calcium diets. In fact, a low calcium diet can be quite harmful by forcing patients to lose calcium from the bones to maintain their blood calcium levels within safe limits. Renal calcium leak is a much less common cause of excessive urinary calcium than increased intestinal calcium absorption.

Patients with renal calcium leak tend to have relatively high blood levels of parathyroid hormone while those with increased intestinal calcium absorption usually have low levels of this hormone. This is because the parathyroid glands located in the neck will secrete high levels of their hormone in an attempt to keep the blood calcium level from falling too low. Medullary Sponge Kidney, described later in this chapter, is more likely to be associated with renal calcium leak. Finally, those patients who are unresponsive to reasonable dietary calcium restriction alone may have renal calcium leak, especially if their parathyroid hormone levels are elevated. Thiazides are the treatment of choice for high urinary calcium levels caused by renal calcium leak.

A Hormonal Cause of Calcium Stones

"Bones, Stones, Moans and Groans" is a rhyme learned by most medical students to help them remember that hyperparathyroidism is associated with two painful conditions: osteoporosis and kidney stones. Both conditions cause the "moans and groans."

Excessive parathyroid hormone (called hyperparathyroidism) is a hormonal cause of calcium stones. The parathyroid glands are four small, soft, yellowish structures located right next to and slightly behind the thyroid gland in the neck. Their function is to regulate the calcium levels of the blood within a very narrow range. This is essential in maintaining proper functioning of nerves, bones and muscles including the heart. Too much (hypercalcemia) or too little calcium in the blood can be very dangerous.

About 3 to 5 percent of all kidney stones are caused by hyperparathyroidism. Calcium phosphate is the main component of urinary stones produced in this condition. Symptoms of the disorder include muscle weakness and lethargy in addition to kidney stone disease. It occurs most often in the 50 and 60 year old age groups. Women are affected 50 percent more often than men.

What Parathyroid Hormone Does

When the calcium level in the blood is too low, the parathyroid glands make a hormone called Parathyroid Hormone or "PTH." This hormone has three functions, all of which seem to have the goal of increasing blood calcium levels regardless of the consequences.

Parathyroid hormone goes to work on the bone and stimulates the bone dissolving cells which increase their activity and release calcium into the bloodstream. This leads to osteoporosis, brittle bones and fractures.

Parathyroid hormone increases calcium reabsorption by the kidney, essentially taking calcium out of the urine and putting it into the blood. (This wouldn't be bad except that the other effects of hyperparathyroidism overcome this one benefit as far as increasing urinary calcium and forming kidney stones are concerned).

Parathyroid hormone causes the kidney to chemically change Vitamin D into its most active form called Vitamin D3 or calcitriol. This activated Vitamin D acts on the digestive tract to increase absorption of calcium and phosphate from the intestinal contents. When the serum calcium level returns to normal and the Vitamin D level is high, production of parathyroid function decreases. The system operates much like your home thermostat regulates the temperature. Usually this works quite well.

However, the problem occurs when one or more of the parathyroid glands continues to make large amounts of hormone when the blood calcium level is normal or even above normal. This condition is called hyperparathyroidism.

There are several reasons why physicians should be concerned about excessive parathyroid hormone levels. If this condition persists without treatment, it will cause excessive loss of calcium from the bones (osteoporosis), dangerously high blood calcium levels (hypercalcemia) and elevated urinary calcium excretion. These high urinary calcium levels are sometimes referred to as "resorptive" because the calcium is " reabsorbed" from the normal bodily storage area: the bones of the skeleton.

The diagnosis of hyperparathyroidism is relatively simple. A routine blood test for calcium, which is recommended for all patients with calcium stones, will detect an abnormally high calcium level and suggest the need for additional confirmatory testing. Any kidney stone chemical composition that is largely calcium phosphate should also raise the suspicion of possible hyperparathyroidism. To confirm the diagnosis, a blood parathyroid hormone level would need to be taken. There are several different varieties of this blood hormone test, but we recommend the "whole or intact molecule" version as being the most dependable. If both the serum calcium and parathyroid hormone levels are elevated, the diagnosis is confirmed.

The treatment for hyperparathyroidism is usually surgery. Any abnormally functioning parathyroid glands must be removed. These are usually located in the neck. Only the abnormal glands should be taken because you still need at least one normal parathyroid gland to properly regulate the blood calcium level. To find a good surgeon for this condition, make sure they have substantial experience specifically in parathyroid surgery. In virtually no other area of surgery is prior experience as important to the final outcome as in hyperparathyroidism.

If for any reason surgery is not possible, an alternative medical treatment is phosphate supplementation which tends to block some of the worst effects of the condition. However, this is often insufficient and surgery should be done at the earliest opportunity.

There are other medical problems that produce high blood calcium levels but rarely cause kidney stones. These conditions include:

- Various cancers, especially lung and breast cancer

- Sarcoidosis and other granulomatous diseases

- Hyperthyroidism (too much thyroid hormone)

- Pheochromocytoma (a tumor of the adrenal glands)
- Steroid excess or abuse

Immobilization and Stone Disease in Space

Anyone forced to stay in bed for long periods of time, such as after a major accident or from a spinal cord injury and paralysis, will tend to lose calcium from the bones of the skeleton. This is caused by the lack of weight bearing on those bones. Bones tend to adjust their strength and calcium content in response to the forces placed on them. The stronger the force, the more calcium is deposited to strengthen the bone. If the process didn't stop at some point, our bones would be too heavy for us to walk. So there is constantly a balance in our bones between the bone making cells and the bone dissolving cells. If very little pressure is placed on the skeleton, such as during prolonged bed rest, the balance shifts in favor of the bone destroying cells because the body thinks there is no longer any need for that much calcium in the bones that aren't being used. The bones end up thin, weak, brittle and likely to fracture. Meanwhile, the calcium that was previously in the bones has now been released into the bloodstream and it eventually gets into the urine where it can create calcium kidney stones.

Many patients on long-term bed rest will require catheters or urine drainage tubes placed in their bladders. These tubes often lead eventually to urinary infections which further increase the risk of stone formation.

Treatment of this type of problem requires some type of weight bearing exercise to force the body to restore the calcium to the bone where it belongs. This is a particular problem in astronauts where weightlessness in space creates exactly the same difficulty. Astronauts utilize special exercises in space using springs and other devices to try to simulate the effect of normal weight on their bones and prevent the loss of calcium. In addition to calcium loss, astronauts in space tend to have lower urinary citrate and volume levels as well as more acidic urine than those same people do on Earth. This is why astronauts are at high risk for kidney stones as happened to one astronaut on Apollo 13 and on several NASA Shuttle missions. (The Russian cosmonauts have had similar problems so it's not political!).

Hypervitaminosis D: Too Much Vitamin D

Hypervitaminosis D occurs when Vitamin D supplements are taken excessively or inappropriately. Vitamin D is essential for absorption of calcium and phosphate particularly during childhood. It prevents rickets and helps maintain healthy teeth and bones. Adults require very little Vitamin D for normal health. There are a few situations where Vitamin D supplements are useful in mature adults such as:

- Pregnancy
- Breast feeding
- Prolonged steroid use
- To avoid Vitamin D related complications associated with some medications
- Selected individuals with osteoporosis

During pregnancy and periods of breast feeding, Vitamin D can increase phosphate and calcium absorption while these two minerals are being shared with the baby. Prolonged steroid use for asthma or arthritis will tend to cause loss of calcium from bone which may be avoided to some degree with Vitamin D supplementation. A few medications will directly interfere with normal Vitamin D activity and might require Vitamin D supplementation in certain situations. Dilantin, a medication used to prevent convulsions, is one example.

Excessive, inappropriate and megadose vitamins should generally be avoided in patients with kidney stone disease. You should certainly discuss this with your physician if you plan on taking any long-term or high dose vitamins for a significant period of time.

Medullary Sponge Kidney

Medullary Sponge Kidney is a benign condition of the kidneys that tends to increase the risk of stone disease. It is diagnosed by kidney X-rays (Intravenous Pyelogram or IVP) and is described as a faint, white blush on the inside of the kidney that is visible only on X-ray. This is caused by dilation of the microscopic collecting tubules of the kidney. It is significant only because people with Medullary Sponge Kidney tend to have kidney stones more often than the general population and may be associated with renal calcium leak. It is unclear if they have a higher incidence of abnormal urinary chemistries than other stone patients. Either way, they should receive metabolic testing and follow specific stone prevention treatment advice just like other kidney stone patients at risk for recurrences.

Milk Alkali Syndrome

This is a condition where there is excessive oral intake of calcium containing foods and antacids. While acid neutralizing antacids are often helpful in preventing most stones, too much will result in various chemical problems in the body that can cause kidney stones of a slightly different chemical composition. Calcium phosphate is often the main ingredient of stones formed in Milk Alkali Syndrome. The obvious treatment is to identify and stop the abnormally high intake of these inappropriate foods and antacids.

Since new heartburn and ulcer medicines were developed that eliminate much of the need for calcium based antacids, the incidence of Milk Alkali Syndrome has decreased. There is a danger that some women who are worried about loss of calcium from the bones (osteoporosis) may be taking too much oral calcium antacids such as "TUMS" or calcium carbonate. For this reason, Milk Alkali Syndrome should be considered (as well as hyperparathyroidism described earlier) in any postmenopausal woman with calcium phosphate stones.

Renal Phosphate Leak

Renal Phosphate Leak is a rare and complicated disorder leading to kidney stones. In this condition, the kidney is unable to keep excessive amounts of phosphate from being lost in the urine. This quickly depletes the blood phosphate level. Low blood phosphate stimulates the kidney to convert Vitamin D into the much more active Vitamin D3. This high level of activated Vitamin D then works on the intestinal tract to increase phosphate absorption from the digested food. Unfortunately, the extra Vitamin D also incidentally increases intestinal calcium absorption resulting in a net absorbed calcium excess. The extra calcium ends up in the urine causing high urinary calcium levels and stones. To make the diagnosis, you would need all of the following four elements:

- High Urinary Phosphate
- Relatively Low Serum Phosphate
- High Activated Serum Vitamin D (Vitamin D3)
- High Urinary Calcium

This can be a very difficult diagnosis to make because few individual testing protocols include all of these elements and it's easy even for an expert to overlook this rare and unusual condition. Fortunately, there is at least one commercial stone prevention laboratory protocol, from Laboratory Corporation of America, that includes all the necessary tests and has computer assisted analysis of the data which indicates to the physician when the four critical elements are present, making the diagnosis quite simple.

Since we can't fix the defect in the kidney directly, we need to treat this condition in some other way. Oral phosphate supplements are the treatment of choice. They are quickly absorbed into the blood so they correct the low serum phosphate that would otherwise stimulate the Vitamin D activation. Persantine (Dipyridamole) has been shown to reduce the urinary phosphate loss and may be helpful in some cases.

Renal Tubular Acidosis

Renal Tubular Acidosis includes four separate syndromes involving abnormal handling of acid by the kidneys. Only one of them, called Type 1 or Distal Renal Tubular Acidosis, is involved in kidney stone production. The primary defect here is an inability of the kidney to make an acid urine. Since the kidney cannot excrete the acid, it remains in the body and makes the blood more acid; hence the name "acidosis." Renal refers to kidney, and tubular indicates the location within the kidney where the problem is found: the microscopic "distal" tubule.

Two-thirds of patients with Renal Tubular Acidosis are adults and seventy percent of them will develop kidney stones. The stone production in these patients can be very severe and lead to kidney failure and even death! When X-rays demonstrate diffuse, multiple stones throughout either or both kidneys (a condition called nephrocalcinosis), Renal Tubular Acidosis should be considered as a possible cause.

Stone formation in Renal Tubular Acidosis occurs due to three specific problems associated with this condition:

- High urinary calcium excretion

- Increased urinary acid levels

- Extremely low urinary citrate

Of these, the very low urinary citrate level is the most significant (citrate is a urinary acid neutralizer and a very important inhibitor of kidney stone formation). The diagnosis is generally made from these urinary chemistry findings. In the past, an acid load was given to patients suspected of having Renal Tubular Acidosis. If they failed to make an acid urine even after a large acid load was delivered into their blood, then the diagnosis was confirmed. Currently, physicians usually just go ahead and treat patients with very low urinary citrate levels with oral potassium citrate supplements. This corrects the problems by neutralizing any excess acid in the blood and relieving the chemical pressure on the kidneys. All the abnormal chemistries return to normal. Unfortunately, we cannot permanently repair the defect inside the kidneys, but as long as the patients take an adequate amount of potassium citrate they will suffer no complications or kidney stones.

Urinary Tract Infections

Infections can contribute to calcium stone disease in several ways. (Urinary tract infections causing struvite or infection stones will be reviewed in detail in a separate chapter later). Should a stone become infected, it may become impossible to get rid of the infection without some kind of surgical intervention on the stone. If a kidney becomes infected and its ureter or drainage tube is blocked, the patient can become very sick and develop blood poisoning or sepsis from the infection. In these cases, drainage of the kidney or surgical removal of the stone is urgent and necessary.

Patients with catheters draining their bladders often get urinary infections. The bacteria that cause most infections release chemicals into the urine that neutralize the normal urinary acid and make the urine very alkaline or basic. This is just what the bacteria need to grow! Under these conditions, it is possible for several types of calcium and struvite stones to form in the bladder or kidneys as well as within the catheter itself which becomes clogged and fails to drain.

Treatment usually consists of antibiotics, increasing urinary volume, bypassing or removing any obstruction of the urinary system and removing any catheters as quickly as possible.

Weight Loss Diets

Many types of diets designed for rapid weight loss can inadvertently increase the risk of kidney stone formation. It is generally considered ill advised to attempt to lose more than 1 to 2 pounds a week. Not only does too rapid weight loss put a strain on several bodily functions including the kidneys, it also makes it harder to maintain the weight loss after the diet period is over.

When weight loss is excessive, the body will tend to break down some of its existing protein instead of just the fat you want to disappear. As far as kidney stones are concerned, it makes little difference if you are digesting protein from a steak meal or excess protein from your own system. There is still a load of protein breakdown products to expel. These breakdown products include uric acid, oxalate, amino acids and ketones. The net result is a substantial increase in the risk of kidney stone formation. Urinary oxalate and uric acid levels increase and the urine becomes generally more acidic, making it easier to form crystals and stones particularly of uric acid and calcium oxalate.

Of the various types of weight loss diets available, some are more dangerous than others for kidney stone formers:

Very Low Calorie Diets will cause a substantial acid load on the kidneys and lead to high urinary uric acid levels. This is a good diet to avoid if you are a stone former.

A High Protein, Low Carbohydrate Diet will lead to high uric acid, oxalate and acid levels in the urine. It also tends to cause dehydration. Some of the high protein liquid dietary supplements advertised in magazines and television fall into this category. Stone formers should avoid this type of diet as well.

A High Carbohydrate, Low Fat, Moderate Protein Diet is probably the most acceptable of the ones presented here. Excess protein is avoided, but enough is provided to prevent bodily tissue breakdown and the release of uric acid and oxalate. The carbohydrate portion should be chosen from foods without high levels of oxalate or much of the benefit will be lost.

Proper weight loss programs require an increase in physical activity and exercise, reasonable nutrition, plenty of water and a long term commitment. Weight loss programs should be reviewed with a knowledgeable physician to avoid unnecessary complications in kidney stone formers.

Overview of Treatment Methods for High Urinary Calcium:

Dietary Measures

Moderate dietary calcium restriction alone may be sufficient to control excessive urinary calcium levels for some patients, but more aggressive therapy with thiazides, phosphates, allopurinol or cellulose and magnesium will be necessary if conservative measures fail. Too severe a restriction of dietary calcium will actually raise the overall risk of stones by increasing free oxalate and other minerals in the intestinal tract that would otherwise bind with the missing dietary calcium. For this reason, severe dietary calcium restrictions of less than 600 mg. per day are not recommended. Reductions in dietary sodium, caffeine and animal protein will also be helpful in reducing urinary calcium excretion.

A high fiber diet consisting of wheat, rice or oat bran has been shown to be useful in reducing urinary calcium excretion by as much as 20 to 33 percent in some patients. These foods bind the free intestinal calcium and possibly decrease the amount of time the food spends in the digestive tract. Surprisingly, no adverse effect has been noted on urinary oxalate. A dosage of 24 grams of supplemental fiber daily has been suggested.

Salt

High levels of dietary sodium (salt) will increase urinary calcium excretion. Patients who already have a problem with elevated urinary calcium are more sensitive than the general population to this effect from high salt intake. Sodium affects the way calcium is handled in the body, primarily by the kidneys. Excess sodium can block the beneficial urinary calcium lowering effect of thiazides and increase Vitamin D levels which will further increase calcium absorption from the digestive tract. For every 100 mg increase in salt, you can expect between 25 and 75 mg increase in urinary calcium. There is also evidence that excessive salt will reduce urinary citrate, an important inhibitor of kidney stone formation.

Lowering your salt intake will not only help reduce urinary calcium levels, but will also help control fluid retention and high blood pressure. Most experts recommend limiting dietary salt intake to about 100 mg per day if possible. This is much easier now that most foods are clearly labeled with their sodium content. Be aware that most restaurant meals, baked goods, soy sauce, salad dressings, ham, corned beef, frozen dinners and fast food like pizza contain a considerable amount of salt. Fortunately, many prepared foods have low sodium versions available.

The Following Five Steps May be Helpful:

- Remove the salt shaker from the dining table.

- Use little or no salt in food preparation or cooking. If following a recipe that calls for salt, use only one-half or less of the specified amount.

- Don't add any additional salt to those foods which already contain it. Salt is routinely added to most prepared or canned foods such as soups, gravies and canned vegetables.

- Reduce the salt content of canned vegetables by draining and rinsing them with water before cooking and serving.

- Use a salt substitute like "Mrs. Dash" or extra black pepper. Be aware that black pepper is high in oxalate so don't use too much.

High Urinary Uric Acid

Uric acid is a urinary waste product the body forms from excess protein such as beef, pork, poultry and fish. Elevated urinary uric acid will increase calcium stone production through two separate mechanisms:

■ First, uric acid will form tiny crystals around which calcium stones can grow.

■ Secondly, the very high acid content will neutralize urinary citrate, an important calcium stone inhibitor. Other urinary stone inhibitors become less effective under these conditions. With less citrate and other effective stone inhibitors available, calcium oxalate stones form more easily. About 15 to 20 percent of calcium oxalate stone patients will have high urinary uric acid levels.

The main source of elevated urinary uric acid in calcium oxalate kidney stone patients is excessive dietary protein. Many of these patients will normally consume one pound or more of red meat, fish, or chicken at a time. The majority of these patients have normal blood uric acid levels and only relatively few will produce high urinary levels without a very high protein diet. Over 80 percent of these patients are men. Calcium stone disease in these patients tends to be more frequent and severe than in stone patients with high urinary calcium!

The first step in therapy is to limit dietary proteins to reasonable levels, but many patients are reluctant to give up their high protein diets. Oral citrate supplements are used next if dietary measures alone are insufficient. Citrate supplementation will neutralize much of the excess urinary acid and help dissolve more uric acid in the urine. Allopurinol (see below) is not generally used in these cases unless the blood uric acid level is elevated, the calcium stone disease progresses or the daily urinary uric acid level is over 1,200 mg which is 50 percent above normal.

Medications and Medical Therapies

Allopurinol

Allopurinol works by blocking the final chemical step in the production of uric acid by the body. Instead, a more dissolvable waste product called Xanthine is produced which almost never forms stones.

Allopurinol is the only medication besides thiazide that has been conclusively proven by double-blinded, placebo controlled studies to significantly reduce calcium stone recurrences. This benefit is essentially limited to those calcium stone forming patients with high blood or urine uric acid levels. These patients tend to suffer from a more severe type of stone disease (see section on Uric Acid). Most of these patients have excessively high dietary animal protein intake and would normalize their uric acid excretion if their diets no longer contained excessive amounts of red meat protein. Bread, rolls, grains and potatoes can be substituted. When dietary measures alone are unsuccessful, then allopurinol can be an effective agent in controlling uric acid production and calcium kidney stone formation.

Potassium citrate supplements can also be used when dietary therapy alone is unresponsive. Potassium citrate neutralizes excess urinary acid, helps dissolve uric acid, increases urinary citrate levels and specifically blocks the formation of calcium stones.

Cellulose (Calcibind)

Cellulose sodium phosphate, a strong intestinal calcium binding agent, will reduce urinary calcium but can cause significant calcium loss if used inappropriately. It must be used together with dietary oxalate restriction and supplemental magnesium. Cellulose has significant side effects and is recommended only when all other methods of reducing urinary calcium levels are unsuccessful. A Calcium Loading Test is considered almost essential before starting long-term cellulose therapy, in order to reliably identify renal calcium leak where treatment with cellulose would be harmful.

A brief clinical trial of cellulose therapy may be helpful in the diagnosis of elevated urinary calcium, but care must be taken to avoid inappropriate or prolonged use except in selected cases of severe intestinal calcium hyperabsorption which is unresponsive to dietary modifications, thiazides and orthophosphates.

Cellulose can cause excessive calcium loss in patients with normal intestinal calcium absorption or renal calcium leak. When used correctly in properly selected patients, the combination of cellulose therapy along with magnesium supplements, a low oxalate diet and high fluid intake will totally prevent new stone formation in up to 80 percent of patients.

Magnesium

Low urinary magnesium may be a contributing factor in some patients with calcium stone disease. Magnesium can act as an inhibitor of calcium stone formation because it binds with urinary oxalate to make a relatively easy to dissolve compound. It will also bind to oxalate in the large intestine and reduce oxalate absorption. In addition, magnesium may increase urinary citrate levels. Some studies have suggested that the calcium/magnesium ratio may be a guide to the risk of calcium stone formation and the need for magnesium supplements. If so, then oral magnesium supplements would be of some help in patients with high urinary calcium but low magnesium levels. The ideal ratio of calcium to magnesium should be about two to one. Under normal circumstances, we only absorb about 35 to 40 percent of the magnesium in our diets. Recovering alcoholics and patients on steroids are most likely to develop significant magnesium deficiencies.

There are only a few clinical studies that actually found low urinary magnesium in kidney stone patients. While one study showed a significant stone prevention effect from magnesium supplementation, other studies failed to demonstrate any substantial benefit. With conflicting scientific studies and no definitive proof that magnesium plays a major role in stone prevention for most people, it's generally thought that magnesium supplements may be helpful in some calcium stone patients with low magnesium levels and high urinary oxalate but is probably not as important as the other five major stone risk factors. (The five major factors are high urinary calcium, oxalate, uric acid, citrate and low urinary volume). Still, magnesium supplements have been shown to reduce urinary oxalate levels. This would make magnesium supplementation useful in cases of high urinary oxalate which has been unresponsive to other measures.

Magnesium supplements can cause diarrhea which may be undesirable in enteric hyperoxaluria patients who characteristically have chronic diarrhea already. Chocolate and nuts are high in magnesium content but they have considerable amounts of oxalate. Potassium magnesium citrate, an experimental form of citrate supplement, would also increase magnesium levels as well as citrate. Clinical trials have shown potassium magnesium citrate to be an even better stone preventive than potassium citrate alone.

Magnesium supplements have been shown to be necessary in stone prevention in combination with cellulose phosphate therapy. When cellulose is used as a calcium binder in cases of highly resistant elevated urinary calcium, magnesium supplementation is required to prevent magnesium deficiency.

Orthophosphates

Orthophosphate supplements are successfully used in many patients with high urinary calcium levels, particularly when dietary moderation and thiazides fail, but they need to be taken often and may have significant side effects. Diarrhea is the most common complication of orthophosphate therapy. This can be minimized by lowering the dosage until the diarrhea disappears and then gradually increasing the orthophosphate supplementation into the usual therapeutic range. Most patients are eventually able to tolerate the orthophosphate supplements.

Orthophosphates will decrease urinary calcium by up to 50 percent through reductions in intestinal calcium absorption and they will increase urinary citrate levels. They are particularly effective in calcium oxalate stone disease when combined with Vitamin B6. Orthophosphate therapy is clearly the treatment of choice for Renal Phosphate Leak where it will quickly correct the low blood phosphate that inappropriately activates Vitamin D in this condition.

Calcium kidney stone formation stops in 90 percent of patients on adequate orthophosphate therapy. Orthophosphate supplements can be used together with thiazide therapy for difficult or resistant calcium stone cases.

Orthophosphate shouldn't be used in cases of struvite or infection stones, high blood phosphate levels, renal tubular acidosis, urinary blockage of any kind, kidney failure or active urinary infection. If the kidney failure is moderately severe, then orthophosphates shouldn't be used. Patients with existing bowel disorders often cannot tolerate orthophosphate therapy. The usual therapeutic dosage range is 1.5 to 2.5 gm/day in divided doses. The neutral salt of phosphate is usually the best tolerated.

A new "Slow Release" form of neutral orthophosphate called UroPhos-K is currently being developed and preliminary results are quite promising. In one study, the new orthophosphate medication reduced urinary calcium by 40 percent without causing any significant digestive tract problems or side effects. There was no change in urinary oxalate, but there was a significant increase in urinary citrate and other important kidney stone inhibitors.

Citrate

Urinary citrate is our single most effective natural calcium stone inhibitor (except maybe for water). It blocks crystal formation and stone production of both major types of calcium stones: calcium oxalate and calcium phosphate. Up to 63 percent of recurrent kidney stone patients may have some degree of decreased urinary citrate. There are a few well known causes of low urinary citrate (hypocitraturia) such as low serum potassium, renal tubular acidosis (described earlier) chronic diarrhea and enteric hyperoxaluria (reviewed in the following section on oxalate). A variety of medications have caused low urinary citrate levels such as thiazides (a water pill), Diamox (a glaucoma drug) and possibly ACE inhibitors (a type of blood pressure medicine). However, the cause of low urinary citrate in the majority of patients with this condition is unknown.

Urinary citrate excretion is usually determined by the overall acid balance in the body. Any bodily function that creates acid or any dietary substance that leaves an acid residue will increase the body's acid load and lower urinary citrate levels. Strenuous exercise or starvation will produce an acid load in the body that will decrease citrate excretion. One example of a high acid residue dietary source would be animal protein like red meat.

Sodium bicarbonate or common baking soda can be used to increase urinary citrate levels. The kidneys will convert the bicarbonate into citrate and excrete it in the urine. The problem with sodium bicarbonate as a therapy for low urinary citrate levels is the large sodium load and the relatively short period of time the medication is effective. For these reasons, potassium citrate supplements are usually preferred.

Potassium Citrate

Dietary supplementation with potassium citrate is the standard remedy for low urinary citrate levels. Available in both slow release tablet (Citrolith, Urocit-K) and liquid (Polycitra K) forms, this medication effectively raises urinary citrate levels and reduces urinary acid. Potassium citrate is particularly useful when given together with thiazides (see section on thiazides below) which tend to decrease both urinary citrate and blood potassium levels. Even increased fluid intake, the cornerstone of virtually every kidney stone prevention program, will inadvertently reduce urinary citrate concentration due to dilution, making this important stone inhibitor less effective.

In selected patients, long-term potassium citrate therapy appears to be extremely effective by stopping kidney stone formation completely in as many as 80 percent of patients and substantially reducing new stone production in up to 98 percent!

Potassium citrate will effectively neutralize excess acid in the urine which makes it useful in the prevention and treatment of uric acid stones. It's usually the antacid agent of choice because of its more uniform effects, ease of administration and lack of sodium.

Acid neutralizing agents such as potassium citrate should not be used in struvite or infection stones. Potassium citrate shouldn't be given together with aluminum antacids or supplements because of the risk of increased aluminum absorption particularly in patients with any significant kidney failure.

The only major disadvantage to the use of citrate supplements is the need for ingestion of relatively large amounts in divided doses. The usual dosage is two or three tablets, three or four times a day but the actual amount should be adjusted individually to maintain the urinary citrate level at or above 320 mgs per liter (or total of 640 mgs per day). Urinary acid levels should be monitored periodically during potassium citrate therapy because excessive acid neutralization may occur which can increase the risk of calcium phosphate stones.

Slow release potassium citrate tablets are convenient, but difficult to digest for some patients. They tend to be more expensive and are slightly more likely than the liquid to have mild gastrointestinal side effects. Patients may notice the tablets in their stool and assume incorrectly that the medication is being eliminated abnormally without absorption. Patients should be aware that what they are seeing is only the wax ghost which carried the medication. The appearance of the tablet apparently unchanged in the stool is normal and doesn't mean the medicine isn't working. If patients fail to adequately raise their urinary citrate excretion despite reasonable doses of potassium citrate tablets, then liquid supplements should be added.

Liquid potassium citrate supplements are more readily absorbed and generally better tolerated than tablets. The pleasant tasting liquid form is also less expensive than tablets, but needs to be taken more often due to its relatively quick absorption. Dissolvable potassium citrate crystals are available in convenient single dose packets which can be mixed with various beverages.

A single dose of potassium citrate in the evening before bed may be a reasonable alternative maintenance therapy for many patients with uric acid stones or low urinary citrate levels, especially if they're having difficulty with compliance or affordability of a more aggressive treatment plan. The body normally produces less acid at night which may help dissolve any early stone crystals. Taking potassium citrate before bed should enhance this natural stone preventing process.

Lemonade can be a reasonable alternative or addition to potassium citrate supplementation. Lemons are extremely high in citrate and it has been shown that 24 hour urinary citrate can be increased by about 200 mg just by drinking 2 liters of lemonade daily. The suggested lemonade is made from 1/2 cup of fresh lemon juice and 7 and 1/2 cups of water which is then sweetened to taste. Lemonade therapy is much cheaper than commercial citrate supplements and is easier to take regularly over long periods of time but requires large amounts to be drunk daily.

Potassium magnesium citrate, which is still investigational, has been shown to increase urinary citrate sixteen percent more than equivalent doses of potassium citrate. It also provides greater stone formation inhibition than existing potassium citrate preparations. When approved by the FDA, potassium magnesium citrate is likely to replace potassium citrate as the preferred urinary antacid therapy for kidney stone patients.

Thiazides

Thiazides were originally designed to treat high blood pressure. They are "water pills" and will increase the urinary volume by forcing the kidneys to make more urine than otherwise. These medication will effectively reduce urinary calcium levels by 30 to 50 percent, but excessive dietary salt (sodium) will block this effect. Thiazides are particularly useful in renal calcium leak, as they take calcium from the urine and return it to the bloodstream specifically correcting the kidney abnormality responsible. When used appropriately for renal calcium leak, thiazides will correct high parathyroid hormone levels, decrease Vitamin D activation and lower intestinal calcium absorption. In other words, they pretty much fix everything!

Thiazides are clearly the treatment of choice for patients with renal calcium leak. They are also well suited for high blood pressure patients with increased urinary calcium where dietary control of their calcium excretion has failed. New stone formation can be completely stopped in up to 90 percent of stone patients with high urinary calcium levels treated appropriately with thiazides. There is evidence that thiazides may help prevent kidney stone formation even in stone patients with normal urinary calcium levels, possibly through a reduction in urinary oxalate.

Thiazides are frequently used to treat high urinary calcium from other causes such as increased intestinal calcium absorption, but the underlying problem would not be corrected and the calcium lowering effect of the medication may be transitory, lasting only a few years. Specifically, thiazide medications may eventually lose some of their beneficial effect when used for intestinal calcium hyperabsorption. Thiazide medications will increase urinary volume due to their action as water pills which could lead to dehydration if the patient's oral fluid intake does not increase sufficiently.

Low blood potassium, low urinary citrate and elevated uric acid levels are commonly associated with thiazide use. Chemically, thiazides contain sulfa and should be used with caution in patients who are allergic to other sulfa medications. About 20 percent of patients must discontinue the medication due to undesirable side effects such as:

- Cholesterol elevation
- Decreased Libido
- Dehydration
- Depression
- High blood calcium
- High blood glucose
- Increased triglycerides

- Lethargy
- Low blood potassium
- Low blood sodium
- Low urine citrate
- Magnesium loss
- Malaise
- Weakness

Low serum potassium and low urinary citrate can be avoided by supplemental potassium citrate. Thiazides should not be used in cases of high blood calcium because they may further increase the calcium content of the blood.

There is an exception to the rule we just stated: that thiazides should generally not be used if high blood calcium is present. A brief trial of thiazide therapy can be useful in detecting those patients with "Subtle or Borderline Hyperparathyroidism." Patients with true hyperparathyroidism will continue to demonstrate high blood calcium and elevated parathyroid hormone levels following a brief trial of thiazide therapy. Normal people will decrease their parathyroid hormone production as the blood calcium level rises.

Lozol (Indapamide) 1.25 or 2.5 mg/day and Naqua (Trichlormethiazide) 2 to 4 mg/day are often the preferred agents for thiazide therapy due to their once a day dosage schedule and reduced side effects. These medications can reduce urinary calcium levels by 30 to 50 percent. Careful follow-up is needed on a regular basis when patients are on long-term thiazide therapy due to the relatively high risk of side effects, electrolyte abnormalities and the possible loss of their urinary calcium reducing effect.

Simple Summary of Calcium Stone Prevention

First, comprehensive metabolic prevention testing is absolutely necessary to fully identify all the medical and chemical stone risk factors present. Risk factors other than elevated urinary calcium (including high uric acid, low urinary citrate, high urinary oxalate and low urinary volume) still need to be addressed and treated.

(1) Moderation of dietary calcium. Too much calcium in the diet is obviously harmful, but too little dietay calcium can also increase calcium stone formation! Roughly 600 - 800 mg. of dietary calcium per day is recommended.

(2) Modify other dietary factors. Excessive salt (sodium) and animal protein should be avoided as well as very low calorie weight loss diets. High dietary fiber will help reduce urinary calcium levels and is recommended.

(3) If dietary measures alone are uncessful in adequately controlling excessive urinary calcium levels and no specific medical condition is identified, then drug therapy will be needed. Effective medications include thiazides, orthophosphates, magnesium supplements and rarely cellulose.

CHAPTER NINE

OXALATE
Getting "Stoned" Isn't What It Used to Be

Oxalate has no useful function in humans and is merely a waste product excreted in the urine and stool. For unlucky farm-grazing sheep, however, oxalate is often a death sentence. When sheep (which had been kept inside barns feeding on low-oxalate hay during the long winter months) were allowed to graze in fields of high oxalate grasses in the spring, they would get sick and even die from the effects of oxalate poisoning.

Chemically, urinary oxalate is a very powerful promoter of kidney stone formation in humans. It has been shown that pound for pound urinary oxalate is about fifteen times stronger than urinary calcium as a promoter of calcium oxalate stone formation.

In the human diet, oxalate is found in almost every vegetable and plant to some degree, usually in the bark and leaves. Its function in plants is to bind calcium and eventually remove the calcium from the plant as the leaf or bark is shed. This often means that identical plants from different geographical regions and even different fields in the same general area will have variable amounts of oxalate depending on climate and soil conditions during their growth.

Stomach acid releases oxalate from food. Most of this oxalate eventually binds to calcium inside the digestive tract and never gets absorbed. Any free or unbound oxalate that reaches the large intestine will probably be absorbed. A decrease in oral calcium intake will result in less intestinal binding of dietary oxalate and increased oxalate absorption. (This is why very low calcium diets are no longer recommended for any calcium stone patient). The daily diet may contain between 100 and 1000 mg of oxalate but averages around 120 mg with most of it being excreted bound to calcium in the stool. In normal people, dietary sources are responsible for about 50 percent of the oxalate that eventually ends up in the urine.

The rest of the excreted urinary oxalate is formed by the liver. The average normal total urinary oxalate excretion is less than 40 mg per day.

There are three types of high urinary oxalate (hyperoxaluria) conditions:

- Mild or Idiopathic Hyperoxaluria (usually due to simple dietary excesses or lack of Vitamin B-6).

- Enteric Hyperoxaluria (a more severe form often involving chronic diarrhea and other intestinal disorders).

- Primary Hyperoxaluria (the most severe of all the types of high urinary oxalate disorders. It's an inherited, genetic condition).

Mild or Idiopathic Hyperoxaluria

This is the most common type of high urinary oxalate and is usually due to simple dietary excesses or relatively mild liver conditions. (Idiopathic means the cause is unknown while hyperoxaluria refers to any elevated urinary oxalate level). Diets high in oxalate content will certainly contribute to an abnormally high urinary oxalate excretion. Excess Vitamin C intake over 500 mg per day can be converted by the liver into oxalate. Lack of adequate Vitamin B-6 will block an important chemical pathway in the liver and cause an increase in oxalate production. A high animal protein diet can also increase the liver's production of oxalate and should be avoided. Finally, a strict low calcium diet of less than 400 mg/ day will increase urinary oxalate due to a relative lack of free intestinal calcium to bind the dietary oxalate and prevent its absorption.

Treatment begins with avoiding an excessively high oxalate, high fat, high protein diet. Tea, chocolate, colas, nuts, green leafy vegetables and berries generally contain high levels of oxalate. Excessive Vitamin C and animal meat protein should be avoided to prevent their conversion to oxalate in the liver. A high fat diet will tend to increase intestinal oxalate absorption. Vitamin B-6 (pyridoxine) in doses of 100 mg. twice a day can help lower oxalate levels in about 50 percent of patients and totally normalize it in about 20 percent. Vitamin B-6 works by promoting an alternate chemical pathway and is most successful in cases of Vitamin B-6 deficiency. Oral orthophosphate supplements can help lower urinary calcium if necessary. Magnesium can bind to oxalate in the intestinal tract and reduce oxalate absorption but is probably more effective when it joins with oxalate in the urine to form a compound that dissolves relatively easily. Intestinal oxalate binding agents (described below) can also be used, but are not generally necessary in the milder forms of this condition.

Enteric Hyperoxaluria:
Antacid Loss, Bowel Disease, Chronic Diarrhea and Fat Malabsorption

Any type of bowel or intestinal disease can lead to an increase in kidney stones. This includes many types of digestive disorders such as malabsorption, Crohn's disease, inflammatory bowel disease, colitis, stomach surgery, short bowel syndrome, jejunoileal bypass, ileostomies and several other specific intestinal conditions. What most of these problems have in common is some form of chronic diarrhea, dehydration, excessive loss of bicarbonate (antacid), fat malabsorption and enteric hyperoxaluria. (Enteric just refers to the bowel or digestive tract and hyperoxaluria means high urinary oxalate).

Dehydration or excessive fluid loss is an obvious consequence of chronic diarrhea from any cause. During periods of relative dehydration, the kidneys will try to conserve as much water as possible to maintain a normal blood pressure. Without sufficient fluid intake, the urine becomes highly concentrated and prone to crystal formation and kidney stones. The remedy is to increase fluid intake sufficiently to overcome the high fluid loss associated with the diarrhea. You should drink sufficient water to produce at least 2000 cc's of urine per day. There is no precise formula to tell you exactly how much water will be necessary, but you can measure the 24 hour urine output and adjust your fluid intake accordingly. Two thousands cc's is exactly two liters or just slightly more than two quarts. If you can fill an empty half gallon milk container with urine in 24 hours, you're probably drinking enough water (see sections on fluid intake and the "IRS Plan").

Bicarbonate (similar to common baking soda) is a form of antacid that is normally excreted by the pancreas to neutralize the stomach acid as food leaves the stomach and enters the small intestine. This bicarbonate is reabsorbed further down in the digestive tract. If there is any intestinal disorder such as an ileostomy, short bowel syndrome or chronic diarrhea there will be a net loss of bicarbonate that has not had a chance to be reabsorbed. This will increase the acid load in the body. The kidneys will try to correct this acid load by excreting more acid in the urine. This makes the urine extremely acid and reduces urinary citrate, a urinary antacid which is an important inhibitor of calcium and uric acid stone formation (when bicarbonate is excreted by the kidney, it is converted into citrate).

Fat malabsorption can cause very high levels of urinary oxalate. Bile salts from the liver and gall bladder normally break up fats in the diet and make them digestible. In fat malabsorption, fat is not digested normally and the bile salts eventually reach the large intestine where they increase the absorption of oxalate. These bile salts also absorb much of the available magnesium and calcium in the small intestine, leaving relatively little to bind with oxalate in the large intestine. If there is insufficient magnesium and calcium to bind

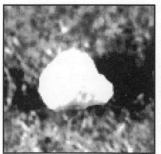

This is a magnified photograph of a calcium oxalate stone. The exterior layers are composed of calcium oxalate and the interior layer of 100 percent calcium phosphate. The stone may have originated as a calcium phosphate stone then collected calcium oxalate and grew. The author was able to pass this stone in the emergency room.

with the oxalate, then large amounts of free, unbound oxalate become available for absorption.

The very high levels of urinary oxalate produced by this process, together with chronic diarrhea, very low urinary citrate levels and quite low urinary calcium is called enteric hyperoxaluria. These patients will absorb much higher levels of dietary oxalate in the large intestine because there are no effective oxalate binding agents, such as calcium or magnesium, available to prevent it.

Interestingly, enteric hyperoxaluria is unlikely if the large intestine has been surgically removed or bypassed, as in patients with ileostomies, because the majority of the abnormal oxalate absorption would occur in the large intestine in this condition. In other words, if the colon is bypassed or missing, then enteric hyperoxaluria generally doesn't occur.

Successful treatment of enteric hyperoxaluria and the more severe forms of excessive urinary oxalate will usually require intestinal oxalate binding agents. The most effective of these is calcium. When calcium and oxalate bind tightly to each other in the digestive tract, neither is absorbed and they both pass out harmlessly together in the stool. This explains why calcium supplements can be used to lower urinary oxalate levels. Calcium citrate is the preferred calcium supplement because of the stone inhibiting effect of the added citrate. Do not use calcium supplements with Vitamin D to help lower oxalate levels because Vitamin D promotes early calcium absorption leaving less free calcium available for oxalate binding in the large intestine. Alternate oxalate binding agents include iron, aluminum, magnesium and cholestyramine. Magnesium is effective but may increase any diarrhea. If necessary, magnesium can be given by injection directly into the bloodstream.

A low fat, low oxalate, low red meat, one gram calcium diet is important therapy in these patients. Vitamin B-6, which works on the liver to reduce oxalate production, should be given but is less effective in pure enteric hyperoxaluria because the excess oxalate is due entirely to increased intestinal absorption of dietary oxalate. If the underlying bowel disorder is due to intestinal bypass surgery for obesity, then serious consideration should be given to reversing the surgery if these other therapies are not successful. Elmiron (see below) can also be used to help block calcium oxalate crystals and stone formation but it has no direct effect on urinary oxalate levels.

Elmiron (pentosan polysulfate) may be of use in high urinary oxalate conditions if other measures are unsuccessful or inadequate. Only limited clinical reports of its use for this purpose are available, but there is evidence that Elmiron can significantly block the formation of calcium oxalate crystals in urine even if it doesn't actually change oxalate excretion. Elmiron is a medication that was originally intended to treat an unusual inflammatory condition of the urinary bladder called Interstitial Cystitis. It's effect on calcium oxalate stone formation was an incidental discovery and has not yet been well studied.

In summary, the treatment of severe forms of high urinary oxalate such as enteric hyperoxaluria in kidney stone patients should include:

- An increase in fluid intake to avoid unnecessary dehydration.

- Sufficient antacids, such as potassium citrate tablets or liquid, to replenish the antacid (bicarbonate) loss, restore adequate urinary citrate levels and avoid an overly acid urine.

- A low fat, low oxalate diet to limit the damage from fat malabsorption and enteric hyperoxaluria. Excessive protein intake should be avoided. Usually 1,000 mg or more of dietary calcium is recommended.

- Oral oxalate binding agents such as calcium citrate, magnesium, iron, aluminum and cholestyramine to help reduce the available free oxalate in the large intestine.

- Pyridoxine (Vitamin B-6) in doses of up to 200 mg. per day which can help reduce oxalate production by the liver. May be less effective in enteric hyperoxaluria.

- Elmiron in severe, difficult or resistant cases, which may help reduce calcium oxalate stones by blocking crystal formation.

Primary Hyperoxaluria

Primary hyperoxaluria is the rarest and most severe form of oxalate stone disease. It's due to an inherited liver disorder and is the most dangerous type of kidney stone disease because of the severe and unrelenting nature of the stone production that can easily lead to early kidney failure and even death. It usually presents in childhood and there is often a family history. Urinary oxalate levels are almost always greater than 100 mg/day in this condition. In children, patients with more than 60 mg/day of urinary oxalate should be suspected of primary hyperoxaluria.

Unfortunately, patients with this primary hyperoxaluria frequently progress to severe calcium oxalate stone disease and ultimately kidney failure. Aggressive combination treatment regimens can control the most damaging effects in many patients. One of the more effective treatments is the combination of high dose Vitamin B-6 at 200 to 400 mg per day and orthophosphates. Orthophosphates lower urinary calcium and the Vitamin B-6 lowers the urinary oxalate level. Magnesium supplements and increased urinary volumes of 3 or even 4 liters per day are useful. Elmiron can also be helpful. Combined kidney and liver transplants may be necessary as a last resort to permanently correct the liver defect which causes the disorder. Fortunately, markedly increased urinary volume, strict dietary measures, judicious use of magnesium supplements together with Vitamin B-6 and orthophosphate can usually control the stone disease without the need for a transplant.

Experimental Therapies for Oxalate

Several experimental treatments for high urinary oxalate are currently being studied. One of these is an investigational drug therapy called Oxothiazolidine (OZT) which lowers the urinary oxalate by reducing oxalate production in the liver. Human studies are currently underway. Early data suggests that OZT could lower oxalate production by about one third.

An exciting experimental therapy involves the use of a beneficial bacteria called "Oxalobacter formigenes." This bacteria is normally found in the intestinal tract where it digests and chemically destroys oxalate. Only about 70 to 80 percent of normal adults still retain healthy colonies of this "good" bacteria in their digestive tracts. It's often lost during antibiotic and other therapies. Unfortunately, once lost from the body, it's very difficult to restore Oxalobacter to the intestinal tract. It also seems that patients with aggressive oxalate stone disease are more likely to have lost this helpful bacteria than the general population. Less than 20 percent of patients with four or more calcium oxalate stone episodes still have normal Oxalobacter colonies in their systems.

Several approaches to this problem with Oxalobacter are being studied at the University of Florida, Gainesville. Stool samples are examined to determine if Oxalobacter is present. If not, experimental therapy can be considered with pills containing oxalate digesting enzymes (chemicals) that were extracted from the Oxalobacter bacteria. Research is being done to find ways to produce the oxalate digesting enzymes directly without using cultures of Oxalobacter which are very hard to grow. Better ways to restore this beneficial bacteria to the system are also being investigated.

This is a very promising line of research which may someday result in major improvements in our treatment of oxalate disorders and calcium oxalate stone disease. Anyone interested in being tested for Oxalobacter should contact the advanced diagnostic laboratory at the University of Florida, Gainesville at 888-375-5227. You can contact Dr. Ammon Peck at the University of Florida at (352) 392-5629 for more information. Also, check out this website: www.ixion-biotech.com. for resources on Oxalobacter formigenes.

An interesting aside, animal studies performed on the sheep mentioned in the beginning of this chapter helped lead to the concept of oxalate digesting bacteria. These bacteria were first discovered in sheep. They help farm-grazing animals digest high oxalate containing grass and plants. Today, before sheep are put out for spring grazing their diets are supplemented with small doses of oxalate to build robust colonies of Oxalobacter.

Gene therapy has the potential for "curing" selected patients with high urinary oxalate. Someday it may be possible to add the gene for oxalate digestion to other bacteria already living in the intestinal tract. This would dramatically reduce the oxalate available for absorption. Unfortunately, such a treatment is years away.

Banana stem extract has been shown to significantly reduce oxalate excretion in rats. Someday, this may be available for human patients with high oxalate problems.

Summary of Treatments for
High Urinary Oxalate

Calcium	Binds oxalate in the digestive tract. Calcium Citrate is the preferred type.
Elmiron	May reduce calcium oxalate stone formation
Increase Urinary Volume	Makes stone formation less likely
Iron, Aluminum, Cholestyramine and Magnesium	Alternate intestinal oxalate binding agents. Magnesium also allows more oxalate to dissolve in urine
Kidney, Liver Transplant	Last resort in most severe cases of Primary Hyperoxaluria
Limit Vitamin C Intake	Excess Vitamin C can be converted to oxalate
Low Oxalate, Low Fat, 1 GM Calcium Diet	Reduces dietary oxalate absorption
Orthophosphates	Reduces urinary calcium. Works well with Vitamin B-6.
Vitamin B-6	Reduces oxalate formation by the liver. Works well with Orthophosphates.

Experimental Treatments

Oxothiazolidine (OZT)	A medication that improves the way the liver handles oxalate. Could help lower oxalate production by about a third.
Oxalobacter	A normal, helpful bacteria of the intestinal tract that chemically breaks down oxalate. Restoring this bacteria if absent or using medicines derived form it may someday be a very effective therapy.

CHAPTER TEN

Why Patients Need to Demand Metabolic Stone Risk Testing

" I n stone disease, everything is measurements. What the laboratory cannot tell you, you will not know; what it tells you in error, you will not correct by using your instincts, your medical experience, or your art; what you take from the measurements directs your treatment. No expense is as unreasonable as years of misdirected treatment, as great as the cost of treating the urologic consequences of preventable stones."

Fredric L. Coe, M.D.

If you haven't had a metabolic stone risk test usually consisting of a 24-hour urine collection and analysis, then you don't have a medical diagnosis for your kidney stone disease. What other disorder of the human body would a physician treat without a specific medical diagnosis?

The success of new technological treatments, like lasers and extracorporeal shock wave lithotripsy has caused some physicians to suggest that evaluating blood and urine chemistry (metabolic testing) is no longer necessary. Adopting this argument is a terrible mistake. Without a diagnosis, there can be no specific medical preventive treatment for stone disease.

In no other branch of medicine would reasonable preventive measures take precedence over surgery. The surgical approach does not totally eliminate pain or affect the rate of stone recurrence. It's relatively expensive compared to the medical preventive approach, and there is always the risk of complications.

Finding the Cause Saves Health Care Costs

Kidney stone disease is a process which almost guarantees progression and recurrence unless the underlying cause is identified and eliminated. This can now be accomplished in virtually every case with appropriate chemical testing, often called metabolic testing, and specific preventive therapies. These preventive measures usually begin with specific dietary changes, with nutritional supplements and medications added as necessary to correct the underlying risk factors for future stone formation.

New advances in the field of blood and urinary chemical analysis and computerized evaluation of laboratory data have made it possible for any interested physician to offer his patients a state-of- the-art kidney stone prevention plan at a reasonable cost. Such a program can be expected to find at least one correctable or treatable risk factor in over 95 percent of patients. While on therapy, most patients will not develop any new stones and existing stones will take longer to grow and thus are more likely to pass spontaneously. Preventive therapy avoids the terrible pain of kidney stones called "colic." Unless you have experienced it yourself, it's almost impossible to describe the intensity of this particular type of pain.

Not all stones are easily removed or treated. An example might be cystine stones which are notoriously difficult to fragment or remove. Any significant reduction in stone formation in these patients would be of substantial benefit. Other patients at high risk would be those with a solitary kidney, renal transplant or any type of chronic diarrhea.

Avoiding Inappropriate Treatment and Preventing Unexpected Complications

Today, non-specific stone prevention advice, such as limiting dietary calcium in calcium stone disease, is no longer adequate. In other words, limiting dietary calcium can actually increase the patient's risk of calcium stone recurrence!

Other problems are discussed in chapters throughout this book, including hyperparathyroidism, hypervitaminosis D, renal phosphate leak, problems with oxalate, citrate, magnesium, renal tubular acidosis and uric acid go undiagnosed and untreated unless comprehensive chemical studies are performed to identify them.

The correct identification of underlying abnormalities will avoid inappropriate treatment and prevent unnecessary complications.

Physicians are primarily responsible for informing their patients who develop recurrent stones about the availability of stone prevention programs. Unfortunately, no significant effort is made to determine the underlying chemical cause or provide specific corrective therapy in many cases. While there may be several reasons why physicians are often reluctant to recommend metabolic evaluations and testing, we believe the patient has to become responsible for demanding certain tests and preventive measures if the physician fails to offer them.

The immediate focus of most physicians is the treatment of any existing stones. This is exciting because physicians get to use all the latest technological gadgets like lasers and ESWL machines to pulverize and remove stones. This is where the emphasis has always been in medical school and residency.

Stone prevention has not always been considered important and some physicians would rather treat new stones as they form rather than stop them from developing in the first place. Some think chemical testing and analysis are too difficult, complicated and expensive. None of these arguments are sound or correct.

Preventing Stone Attacks

Using the latest technological stone removal tools may be fun for the surgeon, but it is unfair to subject the patient to the pain, discomfort and disability of preventable stone attacks. While stone prevention is not emphasized in many training programs, it is the responsibility of every physician who deals with kidney stone patients to become familiar with metabolic testing and preventive therapies. There are a number of post-graduate courses on kidney stone disease and prevention that any interested physician can attend as well as books and medical articles.

Metabolic testing and preventive therapy selection is no longer difficult, complicated, or expensive. Several excellent commercial programs are available nationally that combine many chemical tests in one comprehensive package. Some even offer computerized interpretation and analysis.

The standard of medical care as defined by the National Institutes of Health Consensus Conference on kidney stones, which is as close to a definitive universal standard as we can get in medicine, clearly states that metabolic testing and preventive therapy is in the best interests of patients and should be discussed with any stone patient who is willing to follow treatment recommendations.

Kidney stone preventive testing and treatment is cost effective. The most comprehensive initial laboratory evalua-tion only costs about $400 which is covered by most health insurance policies. By comparison, a single visit to the hospital emergency room for a kidney stone attack costs about $1,500 and a typical hospital admission for a stone is at least $3,000. Obviously the cost increases even more if surgery is required. Lithotripsy costs about $7,500 for each session. The cost of hospital treatment and surgery multiplies by the number of stone recurrences, while the benefits of a preventive evalua-tion and treatment plan remain long after the evaluation is completed. On the average, active stone formers who have comprehensive preventive therapy and treatment can save over $2,000 per year in total health care costs!

Problems with Preventive Testing

There remain some problems with chemical evaluations and preventive treatment programs. There is the potential for side effects from the use of medications and patients may fail to follow all the instructions, particularly over time. The patient must continue the therapy for years even when he or she doesn't feel any immediate pain, discomfort or sickness if treatment is stopped. Frequent follow-up evaluations are required. The initial treatment plan may fail due to poor compliance, lack of proper effect or failure to stick with the treatment plan.

Despite these few difficulties, preventive chemical evaluations and specific treatment plans are clearly in the best interest of patients who suffer from kidney stones. They promote good health, avoid the costs and possible complications of surgery, identify and prevent possible medical complications, and eliminate the pain associated with kidney stones. Fortunately, a lack of availability of the laboratory testing and deficiencies in interpretation expertise are no longer obstacles to obtaining good preventive chemical studies and appropriate, specific medic therapy.

How to Obtain Stone Prevention Testing

If your physician is not interested in pursuing stone prevention testing for you, consult another physician. To find a doctor interested in kidney stone prevention, you can call 1-800- 2-KIDNEYS where a national database of such physicians is kept.

We encourage patients to show this chapter to their urologists. Recognize that you might have to demand prevention testing and treatment. Remember that you are still the consumer and that it isn't the physician who will have to suffer the pain of unnecessary kidney stone attacks. If your physician willingly offers prevention testing, then proceed. But if not, remember that you may have to ask for this help in order to receive it. Below are some of the recommended metabolic testing laboratories. While the blood tests may be performed in the physician's office, the urine is collected as a 24-hour, or sometimes two 24-hour collections and then sent out to one of the specific laboratories below:

Top Six Commerical Programs for Metabolic Stone Prevention Testing

DIANON:

Located in Connecticut, Dianon is a smaller, speciality laboratory that is the newest member of the group of laboratories offering kidney stone metabolic workups. It essentially performs a urine-only examination and provides a graphic outline of the results which is similar to Mission's " StoneRisk" (see below). Additional blood tests are available separately but not as part of the package. Obviously abnormal urine results will receive a one page general summary report about that particular disorder. There is limited consumer information available. Their phone number is 1-800-328-2666.

LABORATORY CORPORATION OF AMERICA (LABCORP):

LabCorp was formed by the merger of two of the larger national medical reference labs: Roche Biomedical and National Laboratories. While they offer a package similar to Mission's (as all of the other programs do) their premier profile called the "Comprehensive Kidney Stone Prevention Program" includes virtually every known potential blood and urine chemical risk factor involved in kidney stone disease and extensive computerized analysis. There is a brief clinical questionnaire that must be filled out by the patient to obtain their comprehensive report, but the result is well worth the extra effort. The excellent report outlines all significant risk factors and provides detailed information, analysis of risk groups and summaries of treatment regimens for that particular patient's stone disease. The program is also unique in that it uses an advanced, proprietary computer "expert" system to analyze the clinical history and laboratory data, including blood chemical abnormalities, instead of the standard urine-only "formula" used by other laboratories. A patient version of their report is under development. This is the kidney stone program we usually recommend. There is limited consumer information available. Their phone numbers are 1-800-222-7566, Ext. 3125 or 1-800-533-0564, Ext. 3124.

LITHOLINK:

Located in Chicago, this lab only does urinary chemistry profiles for stones. Their prices are competitive. Their phone number is 1-800-338-4333.

MISSION:

Mission Pharmacal's "StoneRisk" profile was the first metabolic program available for analyzing urine chemistries for risk of forming new kidney stones. It was commercially released in 1987 and since then has become the leading profile in the United States. The graphic outline is easy to understand

and clear, but doesn't include any blood tests which would have to be obtained elsewhere. Some consumer information on diagnosis and treatment is available. Mission Pharmacal makes many of the kidney stone prevention medications mentioned throughout this book. Their phone number is 1-800-533-3333.

QUEST (NICHOLS):

Quest Diagnostics is one of the country's largest medical reference laboratories. Their Nichols Laboratory in California provides a urine-only profile similar to Mission's at somewhat lower cost. The graphic is easy to read, but only obvious problems can be identified. Other blood tests can be obtained, but are not co-ordinated or analyzed with the urine chemistries. No consumer information is available. Their phone number is 1-800-642-4657.

UROCOR:

This smaller laboratory normally concentrates just on urologists. Their urine-only profile is similar to that of Mission, Quest and Dianon's. Additional blood tests are available but the analysis includes only the urine tests. General educational one page summaries of the significant problems identified are included in the profiles. Their phone number is 1-800-634-9330.

CHAPTER ELEVEN

Women's Special Health Issues:
Obesity, Pregnancy & Osteoporosis

I t's well known that obesity increases the risk for diabetes, high blood pressure (hypertension), heart attack—coronary artery disease—all factors in reduced life expectancy. The effect of obesity on stone disease, especially in women, is not well known by the general public.

Additionally, some women make kidney stones only while they are pregnant and are concerned about the possible effects a subsequent pregnancy may have for developing future kidney stones.

There is also a great deal of confusion about whether women with stones should take calcium supplements, either while they are pregnant or dealing with menopause. Let's take a closer look at these issues.

Obesity in Women and Stones

One major study revealed a link between obesity in women and kidney stone disease. The study, conducted by Dr. Marshall Stoller of the University of California San Francisco, along with Dr. Stephen W. Leslie of the Lorain Stone Research Center and the Medical College of Ohio and others, involved over 5,000 patients. The results revealed a curious and previously unknown connection between obesity in women and kidney stone disease.

The researchers found that obese female stone patients had an increased risk for kidney stone recurrences compared to female stone patients of normal weight. Interestingly, obese men with stones did not demonstrate any similar increase. The researchers interpreted the study as suggesting that differences in calcium metabolism and female hormones (such as estrogen) probably account for this increase in stone recurrence rate.

Another concern for obese patients over 300 pounds (both male and female) is that they may not be candidates for lithotripsy. Such people are simply too heavy for the machine to accommodate, and the shock waves must traverse too much body matter to have any effect on the kidney stones. Procedures performed through the skin are still possible, but are much more difficult since the working distance to the stone is greater, and the pressure on the instruments increases. There is also greater risk of complications from anesthesia and higher infection rates. Obese patients can still receive ureteroscopy and traditional surgery, but the procedure is substantially more difficult and carries greater risks.

In summary if stones occur in obese people, every effort should be made to offer these patients stone prevention testing and treatment once the stones have been eliminated to prevent recurrences.

Should Women with Stones Take Calcium Supplements?

Perhaps the most frequently asked question from women with a history of calcium kidney stones has to do with the issue of calcium supplements. The dilemma is that there are two conflicting health recommendations. To help prevent calcium kidney stones it seems reasonable to limit calcium supplement intake; however, to prevent osteoporosis adequate calcium ingestion is necessary and recommended by many experts. How can we reconcile these two apparently conflicting approaches?

First, we need to know more about the chemistry of the individual patient—which means metabolic testing. Such testing can reveal other problems such as high uric acid levels or low urinary citrate which can then be recognized and treated, and which substantially reduce the risk of new stone formation without affecting calcium intake at all. However, if a high level of urinary calcium is found, then it gets a little more complicated.

It is known that too little calcium in the diet will not only lead to osteoporosis but will also increase the risk of calcium kidney stone formation due to increased intestinal absorption of oxalate. (When there is insufficient calcium in the diet to bind to the dietary intestinal oxalate, the unbound or extra oxalate is absorbed at a higher rate and ultimately ends up in the urine where it increases stone production). This was shown in a research study by Dr. Gary Curhan and a group of researchers at Harvard University. They looked at the effect of a high calcium diet and calcium supplements on the risk of stone disease in women. They followed 91,731 healthy women ages 34 to 59 for 12 years during which a total of 864 women developed stones. This landmark 1997 study found that women with high dietary calcium intake had 50 percent fewer stones than those women who consumed the lowest dietary calcium intake and who then developed the highest rate of new stone formation. The group which took calcium supplements had only a 20 percent decrease in stone production compared to the low calcium diet group.

The calcium supplement group did not do quite as well as the high dietary calcium group for several reasons. They may not have taken enough calcium; they may not have selected the right type (calcium citrate is the best calcium supplement for stone formers), or the supplement may not have been taken at the best time (which is meal time). Of course, remember that this beneficial effect of dietary calcium will be lost if the calcium intake becomes too high.

If the calcium intake is within reasonable limits but the urinary calcium is high, the best solution is to limit calcium excretion in the urine while maintaining an adequate calcium level in the blood and bones (where it belongs). Fortunately, there are medications called thiazides that will do exactly that. Thiazides take calcium out of the urine and return it to the bloodstream. This not only reduces the risk of both calcium stone disease and osteoporosis, but also increases the amount of urine since thiazides are also "water pills" (diuretics). Remember that among water pills, only thiazides and indapamide (Lozol) have this beneficial effect on urinary calcium.

— 115 —

If additional oral calcium supplements are taken, it is strongly recommended that the patient have a test for a urinary calcium after several months of treatment. If the urinary calcium excretion is excessive, then a thiazide medication is indicated. It is further recommended that calcium citrate be used because it is the only calcium supplement that has been proven not to increase the overall incidence of stone disease. (The citrate portion tends to reduce the risk of stone production which might otherwise result from any increase in urinary calcium).

Estrogen, Fosamax and Calcitonin are prescription medications which help increase calcium deposits in the bone as a treatment for osteoporosis. They tend to have relatively little effect on urinary calcium excretion. Estrogen is the most commonly prescribed. This female hormone will help maintain adequate bone mass, but it cannot be taken by some patients such as those with a history of breast cancer. Estrogen has a number of other major effects on the body, most of which are beneficial. However, there may be some undesirable effects as well, so its use should be an individual decision by each woman as she enters menopause in consultation with her physician. Overall, most experts recommend estrogen replacement therapy especially in cases of possible osteoporosis.

Fosamax, a medication that reduces the loss of calcium from bone, or Calcitonin, a bone building hormone usually given by nasal spray, can be used instead of estrogen as alternative treatments for osteoporosis.

In any event, this is a complex issue which needs to be carefully reviewed and discussed with your physician.

Stones and Pregnancy

Lisa developed two kidney stones in her right kidney while pregnant with her first child. After the birth, she underwent lithotripsy. Several stone fragments remained, however, and some eventually grew quite large. Wanting to increase her family with a sibling for little Andrea, Lisa worried about a second pregnancy and the effects it would have on further stone growth.

Actually, Lisa had little grounds for worry. Kidney stone disease affects only about 0.5 percent of all pregnancies, but when present it can be both a diagnostic and therapeutic challenge. There is a normal increase in urinary citrate (a stone formation inhibitor) during pregnancy, which probably explains why more women don't develop kidney stones when they're pregnant. Any medical or surgical intervention has the potential for affecting the pregnancy. If stones are present there is a 40 percent risk of premature delivery. About 50 percent of stones that tend to cause problems during pregnancy eventually pass without surgical intervention.

Stone disease is uncommon during the first trimester, but increases as the pregnancy progresses. The actual incidence of stones is not significantly different from the general female population of the same age. During the third trimester, when the womb is largest, there is very little room in the pelvic cavity. As most pregnant women will remember, their bladders seem to be very small, and they tend to go to the bathroom frequently. Some women reduce their fluid intake substantially just to avoid some of this annoying and uncomfortable frequency of urination. Understandably, any reduction in the amount of fluids consumed increases the risk of new kidney stone formation. A good point to remember is that the end result—a high urinary volume—is the goal.

Diagnosing Stone Disease During Pregnancy

Pregnancy causes a general dilation or stretching of the upper urinary system as the enlarging womb presses down on the bony pelvis. This causes a mild blockage at the entrance to the pelvic cavity and is the reason the urinary system dilates.

This normal dilation during pregnancy can appear very similar to the abnormal dilation caused by a kidney stone (the medical term used to describe any dilation of the upper urinary system is hydronephrosis).

Studies have suggested that serious damage to the baby is likely only at radiation exposure levels approaching the equivalent of 250 X-rays. The average kidney X-ray series or Intravenous Pyelogram (IVP) is only about six films. Still, there is a genuine and realistic concern about exposing the unborn fetus to any unnecessary radiation.

The fetus is most susceptible during the first three weeks after conception. For this reason, any young woman of childbearing age must be given a pregnancy test before any X-rays or other types of scans. Ultrasound, which uses sound waves instead of X-rays, is OK. The next critical period is the remainder of the first trimester.

Ultrasound can often be done first because it carries virtually no risk to the fetus. Ultrasound uses gentle high frequency sound waves and their echoes to form an image. Although quite safe, ultrasound is not accurate or reliable enough to be of much use in the later stages of pregnancy when dilation from the enlarged uterus cannot be distinguished from dilation caused by a stone. Also, most stones are difficult or impossible to see on ultrasound because the average stone is smaller than the maximum resolution and detail yielded by sound images. Most experts feel that a limited X-ray study to establish the diagnosis and help determine the best therapy is unlikely to hurt the fetus as much as an incorrect diagnosis or inappropriate treatment. Therefore, it is cautiously recommended that a limited X-ray evaluation be taken if there is reasonable suspicion of a kidney stone during pregnancy, but not during the first trimester if possible.

Management of Urinary Stones During Pregnancy

Urologists usually try the most conservative measures first. Lots of fluids, appropriate pain medications, and antibiotics are the initial steps. Close cooperation between the obstetrician and urologist are essential for best results. Since 50 percent of any stones present will eventually pass without surgical intervention, waiting is the safest course. Thereafter, every attempt is made to wait until after delivery before resorting to any surgical procedures. But about one third of pregnant stone patients will ultimately require some type of surgery during the pregnancy. The reasons for performing a procedure in these cases are the same as for nonpregnant patients. These include:

- a solitary kidney blocked by a stone

- impending kidney failure

- persistent, severe pain unresponsive to standard medications

- persistent, severe infection

It's possible that the stone attack itself could trigger premature labor—but so could any surgical intervention. Any surgery during pregnancy carries the risk of congenital deformity, abortion, premature labor, low birth weight, and mortality of the fetus. The degree of risk in any given individual is hard to determine. A careful evaluation of the risks and benefits of surgery needs to be done.

Surgical Procedures in Pregnancy

The most reasonable surgical procedures in pregnancy include ureteroscopy, stone basket extraction, double-J stent placement, and percutaneous drainage or nephrostomy. Lithotripsy (ESWL) should not be used in pregnancy because the nature, concentration and type of energy used poses special hazards to the enlarged uterus and fetus.

The safest and least invasive procedure possible should be chosen and this usually means just placing a stent until after delivery. However, stents placed during pregnancy carry a higher risk of getting covered in stone material. (See page 172 for more details about stents). Therefore, they may need frequent replacement and should be monitored periodically for adequate drainage. Any of the other common surgical procedures for stones described elsewhere in this book can be used, with the single exception of ESWL.

Every effort should be made to recover any stone material for analysis. After the pregnancy, an appropriate metabolic evaluation should be made, especially if the patient intends to become pregnant again.

Calcium Supplements During Pregnancy

Pregnant and breast-feeding women are usually urged to increase their calcium intake because they are supplying calcium to the baby. In cases where there is an increased risk of calcium stone disease, either because of previous stone production or a strong family history, it would be wise to use calcium citrate as the preferred calcium supplement, since of all the available calcium supplements, it's the least likely to increase stone formation.

The Differences Between the Sexes

The good news for women is that they get kidney stones much less often than men, by about a three-to-one margin. The bad news for women is that they are more likely to have a metabolic defect such as hyperparathyroidism or renal tubular acidosis, and are more likely than men to have struvite or infection stones.

Women are normally smaller, have less muscle tissue and have tended to eat less animal protein than men. Average urinary uric acid levels also tend to be lower in women, probably due to a lower degree of daily protein breakdown. This results in lower levels of urinary chemical stone risk factors and may help explain why women make fewer stones than men.

Studies show there may be some protective effect against kidney stones from the female hormone estrogen. Urinary citrate is an important kidney stone inhibitor. Women tend to have higher urinary citrate levels than men, but those women who developed stones were also found to have a lower average urinary citrate level than "normal" women and were about the same as men. Many women have a lower daily urinary volume, which is a more common risk factor in women than in men. If they happen to be on vacation or away from home, some women are uncomfortable making numerous trips to the bathroom. This temps them to restrict their fluid intake in order not to void as often. The price for this temporary convenience could well be the accelerated creation of new kidney stones.

Women are also much more likely to develop urinary tract infections (UTI) which can turn a relatively minor disorder into a major, serious problem (for example, if a kidney which is blocked becomes infected and causes blood poisoning).

The following chapter explains in greater detail how bladder infections can lead to struvite or infection stones, and discusses ways to combat these annoying, irritating and often painful urinary tract infections.

CHAPTER TWELVE

Infection Stones (Struvite)

S truvite or infection stones account for about 10 percent of all kidney stones. These stones are mainly composed of magnesium ammonium phosphate and calcium phosphate. Thus, they earn their nickname: Triple Phosphate Stones.

The connection between urinary infections and these types of urinary stones was noted by Hippocrates as far back as 387 B.C. (struvite was named after Baron von Stuve, a Russian diplomat and naturalist).

These stones are always associated with urinary infections. They are created when certain bacteria produce a chemical that decomposes a normal urine ingredient (called urea) into it's chemical components of two strong antacids: bicarbonate and ammonia. Urinary acid normally prevents most bacteria from growing. However, the bacteria which cause urinary infections often neutralize this urinary acid. Without this protective urinary acid, a unique type of stone material called "struvite" tends to form.

Struvite can form only in a very alkaline, low-acid environment. The specific bacteria which can do this have names which sound like science fiction characters: proteus, klebsiella, serratia, pseudomonas, mycoplasma, providencia, staphylococci and some forms of streptococci.

The most common bacteria that cause most urinary tract infections (E. Coli) do not make the chemical that allows the formation of struvite. Other risk factors contributing to struvite stone formation include urinary diversion surgery, recurrent urinary tract infections, neurogenic bladder, urinary blockages, anatomical abnormalities and foreign bodies in the urinary tract such as catheters or stents. Many patients have other underlying metabolic abnormalities. Control and eradication of any urinary infections are essential to preventing struvite stones.

Struvite stones often tend to be large and branched like horns of a deer. They will take up the entire inside space the kidney if they're allowed to grow unchecked. These large stones are also called "staghorn stones" based on their X-ray appearance. As long as there is a struvite stone in the urinary system, it will be impossible to eradicate all the bacteria. Your physician must get rid of the entire stone to remove the source of the infection.

Women tend to get struvite stones about twice as often as men, probably because urinary tract infections are so much more common in females. Struvite stones tend to be found in people older than 60 (compared to calcium stones which are usually found in younger patients). The stones will form again in about 10 percent of patients even after complete removal and in 85 percent of those cases where fragments or remnants remain in the kidney. **If not completely eliminated, struvite stones can cause kidney failure and death in up to 30 percent of patients.**

Lithotripsy can deal with smaller struvite stones up to about one inch in size. Depending on the size and shape of the stone and the internal anatomy of the kidney it may be necessary to use percutaneous (through the skin) procedures to remove the entire stone.

Larger stones may require the use of both techniques. This is called "sandwich therapy" and it has been proven to be the most successful method for treating most larger struvite stones. Chemically dissolving these stones may be possible in some cases but it's difficult to manage, requires prolonged hospitalization, has potentially serious side effects due to absorption of the irrigating solutions, and therefore only works well with small stone fragments.

Preventive Measures

Preventive therapy for struvite or infection stones is based on the removal of all existing stones, eliminating all urine infections, treating any underlying metabolic disorders and eliminating any predisposing risk factors. Catheters should be removed if possible, and urinary obstructions treated or eliminated.

Antibiotics such as penicillin are needed to kill the bacteria. Long-term antibiotic therapy has been used to prevent struvite formation and has even been shown to occasionally dissolve small struvite stone fragments retained after surgery.

Lithostat (acetohydroxamic acid, or AHA) is an effective blocker of the chemical used by the bacteria to create an alkaline environment. Using Lithostat increases urinary acid and reduces new struvite stone formation. Unfortunately, Lithostat produces side effects such as shakiness, deep vein thrombosis, headache, and other significant medical problems which may affect up to 50 percent of patients. A complete blood count is recommended every three months while patients are undergoing this therapy because a very severe form of anemia occurs in about 3 percent of patients.

Lithostat cannot be used in patients with kidney failure, and antibiotics must be used with it since Lithostat doesn't have any antibacterial activity.

When patients are completely stone and infection free, they should be tested for other metabolic stone risk factors which can then be identified and treated. Magnesium supplements, orthophosphates, and urinary alkalinizing agents should be avoided in patients with struvite stones because they may increase new infection stone formation.

Even after all struvite stones are completely gone, it's essential that patients have their urine checked regularly for infection. Doctors recommend a urine test every month for at least three months and then every three or four months for up to a year after any definitive therapy or surgery. Antibiotics are highly concentrated in the urine, so physicians can usually sterilize the urine with relatively low doses of medication. It's often necessary to use antibiotics for long periods of time in patients with persistent struvite stone problems.

In summary: struvite stone patients need to have their stones totally surgically removed. Long-term therapy includes antibiotics to control infections and possibly Lithostat to help avoid new struvite stone formation. Other metabolic risk factors should also be treated when possible. Every effort must be made to avoid further urinary tract infections.

The following chapter provides excellent ways to prevent urinary tract infections.

CHAPTER THIRTEEN

Preventing Urinary Tract Infections in Women

U rinary tract infections are not only uncomfortable, but also potentially dangerous. They can lead to kidney stones as well as serious kidney infections and renal failure. Usual symptoms include urinary frequency, burning, urgency and lower abdominal pain. This can progress to high fever, chills, severe flank pain and blood poisoning in some cases. Nearly 7 million women seek medical help for urinary infections each year and about 250,000 people will develop a more serious kidney infection (called "pyelonephritis") or bacterial blood poisoning (known as "urosepsis").

The basis for preventing urinary infections is to keep the area around the bladder opening as clean as possible with minimal exposure to any new germs or bacteria. Keeping the urinary volume up and proper use of antibiotics are essential.

Wash Your Hands Before Wiping

Wash your hands before you use the toilet or at least before wiping. Wash your hands before you get into the shower to avoid passing germs from your hands to your body near the bladder opening area.

Wipe Front to Back

Always wipe yourself from the front to the back. Don't try to reach from behind because your hand and tissues will pick up germs from the rectum. After bowel movements, clean the area around the anus gently, wiping from front to back. Never wipe twice with the same tissue. Wipe the same way for washing and showering. Do not rub. Soft, white, unscented tissues or "baby wipes" are recommended. A disposable antiseptic towelette may also be used. (Most urinary infections are from bacteria that normally live around the rectum. Any wiping motion that starts nearer to the rectum and then approaches the bladder opening will move dangerous bacteria closer to the bladder).

Take Showers and Avoid Baths

Showers are much preferred to baths. If you absolutely must take a bath, do not use any bubble bath or other cosmetic bath additives. Bath water is full of bacteria from your skin. Sitting in a tub provides the bacteria an easy way to reach the bladder opening area.

How to Wash Yourself

Wash your hands before you get into the shower. Use a fresh clean washcloth. Use a liquid soap because bar soap can harbor bacteria. Do not use a soap for the bladder opening area that has perfumes, creams or other additives. ("Dial" or "Ivory" is usually recommended). Clean the bladder opening area first, before the washcloth picks up any new germs or bacteria. (The same washcloth or hand that washes the rest of your body will pick up dirt, germs and bacteria from your skin. We don't want to move these germs closer to the bladder). Wipe only once with each washcloth. If you need to clean more, use a second washcloth. Try not to over clean this area because washing with soap removes some of the natural protection (mucus) from the bladder opening area. Rinse well and remember to wipe correctly from front to back. The washcloth that cleans the bladder opening area should be used only for that purpose and then laundered.

Douches May be Okay, But Avoid Other Personal Products

In most cases, a vinegar and water douche or a douche with iodine (Betadine) or benzalkonium chloride is helpful if carried out correctly at appropriate intervals. Don't use any feminine hygiene sprays, cosmetics, perfumes, towelettes or similar products in the vaginal area unless approved by your physician.

Use Tampons for Periods

Tampons are advised during your menstrual period rather than sanitary napkins or pads. A tampon will keep the bladder opening area drier than a sanitary pad and help keep any bacterial growth and contamination away.

Avoid Long Intervals Between Urinating

Try to empty your bladder at least every four hours during the daytime while you're awake even if you don't feel the need or urge to void. When you do feel the need to empty your bladder, don't try to "hold it" until a more convenient time or place.

Don't Wear Tight Clothes

Try to avoid wearing pantyhose or tight slacks for prolonged periods. Cotton panties for general use are suggested. Avoid wearing a wet bathing suit for prolonged periods of time. Try to avoid habitual leg crossing. All of these will tend to press the skin folds around the vagina into the body and may introduce more bacteria into the area around the bladder opening.

Drink More Water

Start with one extra glass with each meal. If your urine appears any darker than a very pale yellow, this means you are not drinking enough and should increase your fluid intake. Cranberry juice is helpful, but if you don't like cranberry juice you can substitute other beverages. Follow the suggestions in the "I.R.S. Plan for Increasing Urinary Volume" in this book (see page 141).

Avoid Irritating Foods Like Caffeine

Symptoms of bladder irritation may be aggravated by coffee, tea, alcohol, "hot" spices, caffeine, "NutraSweet,"® chocolate and cola drinks.

Take Vitamin C and Drink Cranberry Juice

Some patients may be instructed to take some additional Vitamin C. This vitamin may help increase your body's resistance to infection. Extra Vitamin C that your body can't use immediately will be released into the urine where it helps block bacterial growth. Cranberry juice may be of some extra benefit in reducing urinary infections. If you don't like cranberry juice, you can get the same benefit from cranberry pills.

Avoid Activities That Increase Your Risk of Bladder Infections

Prolonged bicycling, motorcycling, horseback riding and similar physical activities and exercises may increase your risk of bladder infections. You may need to limit these types of activities. When you do engage in physical activity and exercise, make sure to empty your bladder frequently and drink plenty of water and other fluids. Sexual activity may also increase your risk because it can introduce bacteria into the bladder area.

Take Special Precautions After Sexual Activity

After intercourse, empty your bladder and drink two extra glasses of water. Some patients will be advised by their physicians to take a urinary antiseptic or antibiotic after sexual activity. Make sure you take the medication exactly the way your physician has suggested.

An Estrogen Vaginal Cream May Help Increase Resistance to Bladder Infections

Your doctor may suggest an estrogen cream for the vagina if you have had menopause even if you are already on an oral estrogen supplement or patch. The cream will help keep the tissues around the bladder opening healthy and more resistant to infection.

Take Antibiotics Only As Prescribed By Your Doctor

If your doctor has prescribed a medication to take as preventive therapy, you should follow the doctor's instructions carefully. Be aware that medications may be necessary for up to a year or more depending on the nature and severity of the urinary infection problem. For some patients, a small amount of a urinary antibiotic or antiseptic taken daily will prevent most urinary infections and give the bladder a chance to heal and restore its natural resistance. Other patients may be told to take an antibiotic only when they think they're getting an infection. Take any prescribed medication exactly the way your physician advised you. If you don't remember how to take it and there are no clear instructions on the bottle of medicine, contact your physician or pharmacist.

If You Follow All These Suggestions and Get An Infection Anyway

The guidelines and suggestions listed here will help most women avoid bladder infections most of the time. If you get an infection in spite of these precautions, seek medical help promptly. A urine specimen for examination should be given to your physician. Seek prompt attention for excessive vaginal discharge or other signs of vaginal inflammation and infection. If an antibiotic has been given to you to use for this purpose, you may begin taking it. In some cases, your doctor may request additional tests such as kidney X-rays or an examination of the bladder. Sterilizing your washcloths may be the next reasonable step to take.

Sterilizing Washcloths for Home Use

Your doctor may recommend sterilizing washcloths for washing and personal hygiene to help prevent recurrent urinary tract infections. This extra step is probably unnecessary for the majority of patients with recurrent infections, but for the more resistant or severe case it may be very helpful. Home sterilization of washcloths is only one part of an ongoing program to help prevent these infections. Use only those washcloths purchased for this purpose and remember to wipe correctly, from front to back.

- Wash the washcloths with hot water and soap in your washing machine. If you don't have a washing machine, use soap and hot water in your sink.

- Boil the washcloths in water for at least twenty minutes (optional).

- Take the washcloths out of the water and allow to dry in your clothes dryer.

- When dry, place each washcloth in a separate, sealable plastic bag such as a Ziplock® bag.

- LEAVE THE BAGS OPEN AND DO NOT SEAL THEM CLOSED YET!

- Place the bags containing the washcloths in your microwave. In the center of the microwave, put a large glass of cold water. DO NOT PLACE THE BAGS WITH THE WASHCLOTHS IN THE WATER!

- Put the microwave on High for five minutes and turn it on. Replace the glass (which is now very hot) with a new glass of cold water and microwave on High for an additional five minutes.

- Let the bags cool; close the bags. You now have sterile washcloths inside sterile bags.

This technique will kill the germs and bacteria by using microwave radiation to sterilize the washcloths. Without the glass of cold water to absorb the heat, the bags would melt and the washcloths would burn.

We highly recommend the book "You Don't Have to Live with Cystitis" by Larrian Gillespie, M.D. The revised and updated guide to the prevention and cure of one of women's most stubborn ailments provides important information on newly discovered causes, natural and surgical treatment options, an updated anti- cystitis diet, an explanation of how anti-oxidants can help and a special chapter on how antibiotic treatments can affect your hormones. The book is also useful for understanding cystitis in children, during pregnancy and menopause. Ordering information is provided in the Resources Chapter (page 270).

CHAPTER FOURTEEN

Water, Water Everywhere

E ven Hippocrates recognized the importance of drinking water. The practice of consuming large amounts of fluids has universally been recognized as an important factor in the prevention of kidney stones.

However, time and again we find kidney stone patients who "gag" at the idea of drinking any water, much less "extra" water. Some add flavored syrup to plain water in an attempt to swallow the clear liquid. Others find they must use "flavored" children's straws, or favorite drinking cups. Some have elaborate drinking patterns.

Many don't realize they are "drinking themselves to dehydration" by consuming too little water and too many beverages which rob the body of water.

A recent survey for the Nutrition Information Center at New York Hospital—Cornell Medical Center and the International Bottled Water Association reveals that America's glass is half empty.

The good news is that the average American drinks nearly eight beverages daily such as water, milk, juice and soft drinks. But that is undermined by the nearly five servings of caffeine or alcohol-containing beverages that are also drunk each day. Scientific research shows that caffeine and alcohol act as a diuretic, causing the body to lose water through increased urination.

Most people lose six pints of water a day through the skin and just by breathing. And then there is the need to urinate.

The kidneys contain a nearly 40-mile network of tubes through which fluids filter. The kidneys process 200 quarts of blood a day, straining out waste via urine, then returning the purified fluid to the bloodstream. That's why it is necessary to wash out these filtering tubes hourly.

Fluid intake is the single most important dietary modification for patients with stones. It is the **only** dietary recommendation that applies to all forms of kidney stones regardless of the cause.

In general, at least 8 oz. of fluid should be taken with each meal, between each meal, before bedtime and when the patient gets up at night to urinate. This ensures that the fluid intake is spread out over the day and the urine never becomes too concentrated. At least half this fluid should be taken as water. The rest is up to the individual, unless the diet is restricted in calcium or oxalate. In that case, overdependence on milk, tea, hot chocolate, draught beer and citrus juices must be decreased or avoided.

Also important is that patients with stones increase their fluid intake in hot weather and after vigorous exercise. Just sitting at a desk (considered a routine activity) requires eight glasses of water daily. A brisk walk requires an extra two glasses in addition to the eight. Add a golf session, and an extra four glasses need to be added to the minimal eight. If you're jogging, even more water is necessary.

A hydration calculator is available to determine personal needs at The Brita Products Co. web site at http://www.brita.com/why/hydratecalc.html. The calculator analyzes for weight, travel and dieting.

Without Water—They're Back!

The tiniest microscopic baby stones, called microcrystals, can form objects as large as stones only by growing and combining with other crystals to form a mass of relatively large clumps.

These tiny crystals cannot normally grow large enough to anchor within the five to seven minutes it takes them to pass through the area where the kidney secretes urine. However, when the chemical conditions are right, they can anchor to the lining of the kidney and grow **at leisure to stone size.** These crystals must either anchor themselves firmly in the kidney's lining or be swept away in the urine.

Water is a simple prescription against a sea of health troubles. Drinking plenty of water dilutes concentrated urinary chemicals and stimulates urination which flushes out bacteria.

All You Have to Do Is Micturate (Urinate)

The kidneys filter a remarkable amount of fluid each day—with minimum inconvenience to their owners. Sixty times a day, the body's blood plasma is processed by the kidneys. This means that at any moment, 25 percent of the heart's entire output goes to the kidneys.

The kidneys do much more than filter waste and poisons from the blood. As the body's master fluid engineers, they constantly adjust the body's water, salts and minerals, such as sodium and potassium, thereby regulating blood pressure. Thanks to the kidneys, the total amount of sodium in the body seldom varies by more than a few percentage points, even if you eat an entire bag of potato chips in one sitting. The kidneys produce hormones that help regulate blood pressure and stimulate the production of red blood cells by other organs.

Give Me Water!

One of the best books on this subject is titled *"Your Body's Many Cries for Water—Preventive and Self-Education Manual"* by F. Batmanghelidj, M.D. With this book, you will learn the significant reasons why your body screams for water.

Information within the book deals with water needs at different stages of life, the important properties of water, the initially silent compensation mechanisms associated with dehydration, the effects of drinking alcohol and diet sodas, why the color of urine is important, the impact of the health care system, and our responsibilities as patients.

Dr. F. Batmanghelidj, a graduate of St. Mary's Medical School of London University, and a native of Iran conducted his research in America.

"Your Body's Many Cries for Water " encourages patients not to "drown" in water in an attempt to reverse chemical interac-

Kidneys At Work

Blood plasma processed in one day by the kidneys: 180 liters or about 200 quarts.

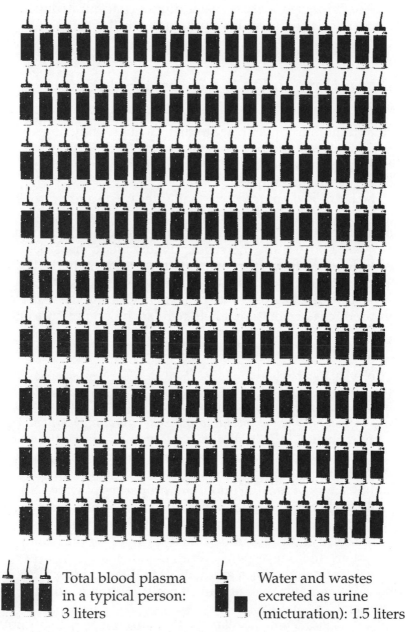

Total blood plasma in a typical person: 3 liters

Water and wastes excreted as urine (micturation): 1.5 liters

Reprinted with permission: FDR Publications, Allentown, Penn. 1993 tions. Dr. Batmanghelidj explains, "the cells of the body are like sponges, and will take some time before they become better hydrated."

Dr. Batmanghelidj recommends that patients drink an absolute minimum of six to eight 8-ounce glasses of water a day.

This book should be required reading for all kidney stone patients, as well as many others who suffer from disease or health ailments..

Health experts agree that people need to drink water even before they feel thirsty, particularly while dieting or exercising. People who exercise regularly or live in a hot climate will need to drink even more than eight glasses daily to replace what they lose through excess perspiration—as much as a quart or two more than usual. Experts advise people should not wait until they're thirsty to drink; that's a signal they're already low on water. The body loses more water than usual through perspiration in hot weather. Thirst, the body's signal to replace that water, often isn't as good an indicator as is needed, particularly in older people. The thirst mechanism becomes less efficent with age. Juices, fruits, vegetables, and caffeine-free soft drinks can provide some of the daily water needed. Except for grapefruit juice which, according to a Harvard study, raised the risk of kidney stones 44 percent!

Patients with kidney stones need to develop the habit of drinking lots of water—for the rest of their lives. When the urine becomes concentrated, the minerals it contains tend to solidify into everything from gravel to full-blown stones. Sometimes half the day passes before one feels the need for fluids. No light goes on signaling: "time to drink water." How does one increase fluid intake?

Physicians and dietitians recommend that patients schedule time to drink glassfuls of water throughout the day. For example, drink a glass of water every hour in front of the computer at work and by day's end the daily requirement will be met.

Choose foods that contain high amounts of water—fruits and vegetables such as lettuce (96 percent), watermelon (93 percent), green beans (88 percent), broccoli (89 percent) and carrots (88 percent).

If plain water is boring, add a squeeze of lime, lemon or orange. Other ways to incorporate drinking water into daily activities include: keep a glass or jug readily available on your desk at work, carry a bottle of water with you as you drive to work or run errands, try filling a half-gallon jug with water and putting it in the refrigerator. You should finish it off by the end of the day.

For more information about water, try these sources:

- American Dietetic Association: www.eatright.org.

- International Bottled Water Association (800) 928-3711; www.bottledwater.org.

- FDA Center for Food Safety and Applied Nutrition (800) 332- 4010.

- EPA Drinking Water Hotline (800) 426-4791.

But I am Drinking Fluids!

Many patients who develop kidney stones think that as long as it's liquid, their beverage will benefit them. However, according to a study published in Urology by Gary H. Weiss, M.D., Ph.D., Patrick M. Sluss, Ph.D., and Charles A. Linke, M.D., cola-flavored carbonated beverages may actually enhance kidney stone formation.

Marked changes took place in the urine of patients who drank large quantities of cola-flavored carbonated beverages. These beverages possibly favor stone formation because of their high acid ash, high sugar, and/or high oxalate content.

The three participants who succeeded in drinking three quarts of cola per day showed an average of 8.3 mg. increase in their 24-hour urinary excretion of oxalate, a promoter of stone formation. Citrate (an inhibitor for kidney stones) decreased an average of 122 mg.

Coca-Cola® Says "Drink Me!"

While the test subjects were instructed to consume three quarts of Pepsi-Cola® per day for 48-hours, many people do not drink that amount in any one day. I contacted The Coca-Cola® Company regarding that study. Dr. Debra Ponder, manager for nutritional sciences said cola beverages have never been demonstrated in a controlled study to contribute to kidney stones.

She stated that one of the most recent and largest studies addressing this issue came from the Harvard School of Public Health. One of the researchers, Dr. Walter Willett, is internationally known for his studies on dietary intake as it relates to various disease states. This is the same study which found high dietary calcium intake decreased the risk of kidney stones.

The study found "no association between the consumption of sugared cola(s) and risk for kidney stones."

Even so, many doctors choose to be conservative in their recommendations to patients. If even a slight association exists between a particular disease and some dietary factor, patients are often advised to avoid that dietary food. With kidney stones however, one has to be careful when restricting fluids since dehydration is unquestionably linked to an increased riøsk for the development of kidney stones.

Most physicians tell their patients that coffee and caffeinated soft drinks are not good replacement fluids because the caffeine acts as a diuretic (increases the production of urine) and causes even more loss of fluids. In addition to coffee and cola, tea and chocolate are common sources of caffeine and oxalates. The caffeine content in coffee depends on the variety of coffee bean and how it was ground and brewed. One cup of brewed coffee contains about 115 milligrams of caffeine. A cup of brewed tea contains about half as much. Soft drinks are a major caffeine source for children and adolescents because manufacturers often add caffeine to these beverages. On average, caffeinated soft drinks supply about 45 mg. of caffeine per serving. A cup of hot chocolate contains only about 5 mg. of caffeine.

Alcohol, as anyone who has downed a beer or two can attest, has the same diuretic effect as coffee and colas containing caffeine. Alcohol may add to the risk of stone formation. Recent evidence suggests a correlation between alcohol consumption and levels of urinary calcium and uric acid. Beer (particularly draught beer) is known to contain oxalate and guanosine which is metabolized to uric acid in the body. Alcohol should therefore be consumed in moderation by people with calcium stones.

How to Achieve Water Balance

One gauge of whether you are in 'water balance' is to simply watch the color of your urine. If it is dark and yellow, you are not drinking enough. The urine should be pale and watery. It will have more color in the early morning due its normal increase in concentration overnight but during the day urine should be almost clear.

People who eat large amounts of protein each day require even more water to rid the body of dissolved protein break-down products such as uric acid. Water helps dilute the food chemicals that cause stones to develop, helps the kidneys work better and reduces the risk for urinary infections.

What About Mineral Water?

Researchers in South Africa recently studied the benefits of drinking mineral water and the effects it had on patients who are stone formers. Their findings suggest that male stone formers in particular who drank a bottled, French mineral water containing high concentrations of calcium and magnesium may help reduce their risk for kidney stones.

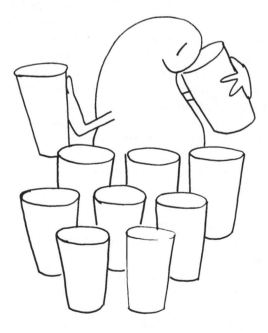

Lead researcher Allen Rodgers, Ph.D. reports the study linked three key factors of high fluid intake, magnesium ingestion and increased dietary calcium as combined ways to reduce calcium oxalate stones risk. Study participants drank a French mineral water, Vittel Grande Source® which contained calcium (202 ppm) and magnesium (36 ppm).

Unfortunately, the particular mineral water used in the study is not available in the United States. Patients who are keen to try this kind of therapy should therefore attempt to find a mineral water that is rich in calcium and magnesium with concentrations approaching those found in Vittel Grande Source®.

Previously, a study of over 45,000 male subjects in the United States by Dr. Gary Curhan showed that a high dietary intake of calcium reduced the risk of calcium oxalate kidney stones. In addition, it has been known for some time that magnesium is an inhibitor of this type of stone.

Several studies have addressed the question of whether tap water (particularly hard and soft water) bears any relationship to the incidence of kidney stones or not. The results of those investigations have been inconclusive.

Eighty patients participated in the study, which was published in *Urologia Internationalis*, 1997. Twenty subjects from each of the following groups: healthy males, healthy females, male calcium oxalate kidney stone formers and female calcium oxalate kidney stone formers were tested. The healthy subjects had no prior history or indications of kidney stones and were between the ages of 20 and 48 years. All of the stone formers were from 25 to 55 years old and they all had suffered the spontaneous passage or surgical removal of a urinary stone during the proceeding six months.

The group which benefitted most from drinking tap water or mineral water was the male stone formers. Mineral water favorably altered nine risk factors (citrate excretion, magnesium excretion, urinary volume, relative supersaturations of calcium oxalate, uric acid and calcium phosphate, oxalate:magnesium ratio, calcium oxalate metastable limit, oxalate:metastable limit ratio and calcium:metastable limit ration).

While male stone formers also benefitted from tap water ingestion, this did not occur to the same extent as that achieved by mineral water. Male controls also benefitted from the mineral water; however the mineral water was found to be more beneficial than the tap water. Healthy female controls benefitted from both drinking mineral water and tap water but the effects of the mineral water on female controls were far superior. Female stone formers were the least affected by drinking either mineral or tap water; however, the mineral water was probably more beneficial than tap water.

In South Africa, kidney stones occur in 15 percent of caucasian males and 6 percent of caucasian females. The Black population is relatively immune but stone disease is starting to occur among urban Blacks. It is unclear whether the immunity is due to dietary differences, a disparity in fluid intake, handling of solute, and/or the presence or absence of inhibitors and promoters of stone formation. Thus, about 200,000 stones occur in South Africa every year and these cost the country in excess of $20,000,000 annually.

Water is our best and healthiest beverage. The following chapter includes some creative ways of maintaining adequate water throughout the day and night. Here's a toast to Hippocrates!

CHAPTER FIFTEEN

The IRS* Plan for Increasing Urinary Volume

After passing his first kidney stone, a patient who had just spent five years in the military quipped that the Army should change its slogan to "Pee All That You Can Pee!"

As the soldier's quip indicates, an adequate urinary volume is absolutely essential for the prevention of kidney stones and recurrent urinary tract infections. The average 24-hour urinary volume is about 1300 cc's a day. Patients with kidney stones or recurrent urinary infections should produce about 2000 cc's, or a little more than two quarts each day. A low urinary volume significantly increases the concentration of calcium, salts and other minerals predisposed to kidney stone formation and irritation of the bladder.

A high urinary volume can reduce the bacterial count and actually cure mild bladder infections by purging the bacteria faster than they can multiply. The simplest, most effective way to achieve this is to drink enough fluids. At least half of any increased oral fluid intake should be water. This is what the body was designed for.

This is often difficult for many patients. The "IRS Plan" for increasing fluid intake and urinary output may help.

*Internal Renal Stone

(IRS) Plan for Increasing Urinary Volume

The "IRS plan" (Internal Renal Stone) may be the easiest way to change your fluid intake significantly. The plan calls for you to drink something called a "tax" every time you enter a room or change an activity. Thus there's a "kitchen tax," a "bathroom tax," a "meal tax," a "medication tax," a "night-time bathroom use tax," a "penalty tax," a "restaurant tax," a "snack tax," a "summertime tax," a "time tax," a "work tax," and a "water fountain tax!" You should add as many "taxes" as necessary to reach and maintain the desired level of urinary volume.

Each "tax" in the plan consists of a 4 to 8 oz. glass of water or other beverage. Use bottled water if you don't like the taste of your local tap water. Choose an alternate beverage that you like. Lemonade, made with real lemon juice, is highly recommended because it's rich in citrate, which helps prevent stones. We suggest that you start at just 4 ounces per glass and let your body adapt to the increased fluid intake.

Make sure that good drinking water is readily available at work and at home. For example, place a bottled water dispenser in your bathroom. Keep a thermos or sport bottle of water near you at work so you can easily grab a quick drink.

Depending on your individual tolerance and metabolism, your system will gradually adjust to the increased fluid, and you will become thirsty if you fail to keep your fluid intake up. The adjustment usually takes about four to six weeks.

The Taxes:

KITCHEN TAX
One glass whenever you've entered your kitchen and wish to leave.

MEAL TAX
One extra glass with each meal except if you eat at a restaurant where you will need to drink two extra glasses of water.

MEDICATION TAX
One full glass with any medication taken during the day.

NIGHT-TIME BATHROOM USE TAX
One glass whenever you get out of bed to go to the bathroom at night. If you're already up anyway, you might as well add that extra glass of water.

PENALTY TAX

If you eat or drink a food item you've been instructed to avoid or limit, you must drink at least two extra glasses of water.

RESTAURANT TAX

When you eat at a restaurant you need to double the meal tax to two glasses. (This is because restaurant food is high in salt which causes you to retain water).

SNACK TAX

At least one extra glass if you have a snack between meals or at bedtime.

SUMMERTIME TAX

During the summer months or whenever the outside temperature is over 75 degrees, you must double all the other taxes!

TIME TAX

One glass if you've managed to avoid all the other taxes for at least two hours.

WATER FOUNTAIN TAX

Whenever you pass a water fountain, you are required to take a drink consisting of at least 10 swallows.

WORK TAX

One glass whenever you leave your desk or designated work area.

Keep a sports bottle with you in the car. If you drive long distances, take a drink every 100 miles and every time you pass a rest stop or service center even if you don't stop.

Substitute high fluid content desserts in place of pastries, cookies and cakes. Frozen ices, sherbet, melons and other fruits are recommended.

Maintain the humidity level in both home and workplace between 40 and 45 percent to minimize fluid loss through the skin and through respiration.

Limit your salt intake. Salty food can cause you to retain fluid and make the urine more concentrated. Avoid heavily seasoned and processed foods.

If these suggestions fail to increase your urinary output sufficiently, a "water pill" (or a diuretic) can be used as a last resort. This will force an increase in urinary volume but can cause mineral and salt imbalance in the blood, plus a number of other complications. Failure to increase fluid intake while taking a water pill could lead to dehydration.

It's rarely necessary to resort to all of these measures to increase urinary output adequately. Check your progress by measuring your urinary volume and add as many "taxes" as necessary to achieve an optimal total. This will reduce your risk of recurrent infections and particularly of kidney stones.

Remember, without an adequate fluid volume no other stone prevention therapies are likely to work.

CHAPTER SIXTEEN

Cystine & Cystinuria:
The Stone Disease You Inherit

Cystine stones are some of the hardest materials to dissolve, yet they often affect the softest, most lovable people in our lives: our children. If you or your children don't have cystine stones, then you probably should skip this chapter, because it will be directed just to people with a personal or family history of cystine stone formation.

All proteins are made up of long and complicated strings of chemical compounds called amino acids. There are only twenty-two amino acids but the number and sequence of these amino acids are what makes one protein different from another. Think of it as using letters to make sentences, paragraphs, and books, yet there are only 26 letters of the alphabet. In this way a relatively small number of amino acids can make any kind of protein whether liver, heart, muscle, or skin.

One of these amino acids is called cystine. This is important in people with an abnormality in the intestinal absorption and urinary excretion of cystine which can cause stones.

The presence of excessive amounts of cystine in the urine is called cystinuria. Cystinuria is a genetic disorder of defective amino acid transport in the kidneys and gastrointestinal tract. It's inherited from your parents.

Up to 5 percent of the population carry one copy of the gene but don't usually form stones although their urinary

THE KIDNEY STONES HANDBOOK

cystine level may be somewhat higher than normal. Children can get cystinuria if they inherit one copy of the defective gene from each parent. Only people who inherit two copies of the cystinuria gene will get the disease. This happens to about one person in 20,000. Men and women are affected equally, but men seem to have more severe problems.

In cystinuria, large amounts of cystine are excreted into the urine. Actually, large quantities of three other amino acids called ornithine, lysine and arginine are also excreted in the urine, but they don't form stones.

Cystine is the most significant amino acid clinically because it is the least dissolvable. Cystine forms moderately opaque branched stones, often with small stone satellites, which tend to be extremely hard and tough.

Cystine constitutes only about one to two percent of all adult urinary stones, but up to 8 percent of all pediatric stones. Therefore, a screening for cystinuria should be done in every pediatric patient who has kidney stones, especially if the stone material is not available for analysis or if there is a family history of stones.

Cystine tends to dissolve more easily in water as the acid content decreases. Acid level is measured by pH. The lower the pH, the greater the acid content of the liquid being tested. A pH of 7.0 is considered neutral like water. Urine is normally slightly acid with a pH between 5.0 and 7.

We can dissolve about 300 mg of cystine in one liter of water at a pH of 7.0 but 600 mg of cystine will dissolve at a pH of 7.5 and up to 1000 mg at a pH of 8.0.

Therefore, it would seem reasonable to try to take antacids (like potassium citrate) which will neutralize urinary acid and increase the pH so that more cystine will dissolve.

This is in fact the case—but there is a problem. As the pH rises to 8.0 and above, a new type of stone material called calcium phosphate tends to form. This calcium phosphate will not dissolve, and it can coat the cystine stones like paint, making it impossible to dissolve them. The best compromise solution is to do three things:

1. Increase the urinary volume to 3,000 or even 4,000 cc's per day by increasing the consumption of water and other beverages. This is much higher than for most stone formers, but cystine patients are special and need this extra fluid.

2. Take antacids like potassium citrate and monitor the urinary acid content (pH) so that we increase the dissolving power of the urine without risking the formation of calcium phosphate. This would mean an optimal pH of about 7.5 without going up to 8. By monitoring the pH several times a day with the use of pH testing papers (available in most craft centers) or through pharmacies as dip-sticks, and spreading out the citrate supplements, it is possible to keep the urinary acid level optimized to make it as easy as possible for the cystine stones and crystals to dissolve and stay in liquid form. Potassium citrate is the preferred antacid for this purpose because it works over a long period of time and doesn't add any sodium. It's also available as both a liquid (Polycitra-K) and a tablet (Urocit-K) by doctor's prescription.

3. Limit sodium (salt) intake which can also reduce cystine excretion.

Cystine stone-formers usually excrete more than 400 mg of cystine daily, whereas normal excretion is less than 30 mg per day. People who have only partial cystinuria, (that is, they have only one copy of the abnormal gene), excrete less than 400 mg of cystine per day and rarely form stones.

Cystinuria patients often have a positive family history and may demonstrate characteristic hexagon-shaped cystine crystals in their urine. The diagnosis of cystinuria is suggested by a daily urinary cystine excretion in excess of 150 mg and is confirmed by chemical analysis of the stone material. It should be noted that up to 40% of the stones passed by cystine stone formers may contain calcium so a complete metabolic evaluation should still be performed.

Cystine: Therapeutic Measures

Initial Therapy

Patients with cystine stones require lifelong therapy to reduce the formation of cystine stones. Medication must be taken several times a day and urinary volume and pH monitored frequently. It must be recognized by both patients and physicians that even with optimal therapy, it is still possible for patients to occasionally form cystine stones.

Initial treatment of cystinuria consists of significantly increased urinary fluid output, dietary sodium restriction, and urinary alkalinization (antacid therapy).

Increased fluid treatment requires expanding the urinary volume to three or even four liters (a liter is slightly more than a quart) a day to maintain a urinary cystine concentration of less than 150 mg per liter and a very dilute urine. This will require a very substantial oral fluid intake of over three to four quarts a day. In the more severe cases of cystinuria, patients should be instructed to wake up at night to drink additional fluids. Urinary acids must be completely neutralized with antacids because cystine dissolves best when the urine is slightly alkaline.

A reduction of dietary sodium intake will significantly decrease cystine excretion in cystinuria patients. Dietary sodium restriction alone can reduce urinary cystine excretion by over 150 mg per day! Therefore, it is strongly recommended that every cystinuria patient be placed on a low sodium diet.

Urinary pH should be maintained at about 7.5, which can be done with various antacids. (For informatin about pH and urinary acids, see page 70.) The most common agents are potassium citrate and baking soda (sodium bicarbonate) in various forms. Overly aggressive treatment with these agents should be avoided, however, since they may produce calcium phosphate which forms its own stones or covers existing cystine stones. Potassium citrate is usually the preferred agent due to its more uniform effect. It also delivers less of a sodium load than bicarbonate.

Acetazolamide (Diamox), a drug normally used for glaucoma, can reduce urinary acid excretion and promote continuous acid neutralization, especially overnight. Such agents should be used cautiously because they can promote calcium phosphate formation.

Allopurinol, a prescription medication, can be used to reduce uric acid excretion and assist with acid neutralization. Lowering dietary acid ash will help limit urinary acids as well. Patients should regularly monitor their urinary pH, especially at night, to be certain it remains within the recommended guidelines and modify the dosage of antacid medications as needed on a daily basis.

Urinary cystine can be lowered by limiting dietary methionine, a cystine precursor, but this results in a largely vegetarian diet which will severely limit protein intake and is usually unpalatable. Most patients cannot stick to such a diet. Significant protein restriction would be dangerous in children. As noted previously, a low sodium diet helps in reducing cystine excretion. High urinary cystine that is resistant to these measures requires more aggressive medical therapy.

In general, mild dietary restrictions, together with increased fluid intake and urinary antacid therapy, will be sufficient in most cystinuria patients whose daily cystine output is less than 500 mg. If these measures are unsuccessful or if the 24-hour urinary cystine is greater than 500 mg, additional medical therapy will be necessary.

Medical Therapy For Resistant Cystinuria

The goal of medical therapy is to reduce urinary cystine to an optimal concentration of less than 200 mg per liter. In addition to all the previously mentioned treatments, the following medications can be used:

Penicillamine (Cuprimine) reduces cystine excretion by reacting with it to produce a complex compound which is more soluble than cystine alone. Penicillamine will effectively reduce cystine stone formation and has been shown to dissolve existing cystine stones, although this may take a year or longer. Penicillamine doesn't appear to lose any effectiveness even when used for long-term therapy. Unfortunately, potentially serious side effects from penicillamine are quite common, affecting up to 50% or more of patients who find they are unable to tolerate the medication.

These side effects include joint pain, skin rashes, retinal bleeding, swelling of the lymph nodes, kidney disease, impaired wound healing, and loss of taste. When initiating therapy, it's recommended that only a small dose be used. Adjustments are then made based on tolerance to the medication and urinary cystine levels. Penicillamine therapy will produce a Vitamin B-6 (pyridoxine) deficiency which is preventable by taking supplemental 50 mg tablets of Vitamin B-6 twice a day. Side effects from the penicillamine therapy are much less common if the total dosage is less than 1000 mg per day, which is sufficient to help dissolve about 300 mg of urinary cystine.

Alpha-MPG (Thiola) appears to be equally as effective in reducing cystine excretion as penicillamine and has a similar mechanism of action. But its side effects are less common and not quite as severe. Unlike penicillamine, Alpha-MPG may lose some of its activity over time, but it doesn't cause Vitamin B-6 deficiency. Side effects include increased susceptibility to bleeding, muscle weakness, joint pain, diminished taste, and intestinal problems. The medication is given three times a day either one hour before or three hours after meals. The exact dosage depends on the urinary cystine excretion level. Periodic adjustments will be necessary.

A new cystine binding agent called **Bucillamine (Rimatil)** is currently under investigation.This new medication is similar to penicillamine but has two cystine binding sites instead of one. This should make it effective at a lower dose than penicillamine and therefore safer and better tolerated. Preliminary results are encouraging, but additional studies are needed before it will be available for general use.

Captopril, a commonly used high blood pressure medication, reportedly forms a dissolvable compound with cystine which is 200 times more soluble than cystine alone. Captopril is very well tolerated and side effects are minimal, but its effectiveness in cystinuria is still unproven. In view of its relative safety, captopril may well be worth a try, especially in high blood pressure patients, before resorting to more toxic agents.

N-acetylcysteine (NAC) has recently been recommended by some experts as the treatment of choice for symptomatic cystinuria patients. In one study involving 33 cystinuria patients followed for 25 years, NAC was found to be as effective as penicillamine and thiola (Alpha-MPG) but without the serious side effects associated with these two medications. NAC is available in health food stores, not pharmacies, as a 600 mg. capsule which should be taken four times a day. Antacid therapy, dietary sodium restriction and oral fluid intake optimization are still required with NAC therapy.

In rare cases of severe kidney failure, cystinuria can be cured by a kidney transplant. The new kidney does not have the cystinuria defect, and this eliminates the disorder.

The Cystinuria Support Network, found on page 264, is a wonderful resource for locating urologists familiar with this type of kidney stone. The Network provides newsletters and information on the latest medical advances on this difficult stone problem and is staffed by compassionate people who "have been there."

CHAPTER SEVENTEEN

Gail's Lithotripsy:
The Second and Third Experiences

I went shopping at Macy's department store only three days after my second lithotripsy procedure in the summer of 1992.

I don't know if the flashing neon lights, the smell of new clothes, or the sound of the cash register bells contributed to my overall good health, but within a few hours of the Macy's visit, I started to pass most of the larger stone fragments.

Maybe shopping can do wonders for your personal health! If you had seen me a few days prior to the procedure, you would have met a very anxious patient. I like to joke that in addition to kidney stones I inherited a worry gene from my father's side of the family.

During a "pre-op" visit with my urologist, I viewed a video explaining what to expect during lithotripsy and what the recovery would be like.

I related closely to the patient in the video. She was driving along the California coastline with its dramatic scenes of the wild Northern coast and its famous hairpin turns. I have always loved the ocean, and yet during the previous three years on every trip to the coast, along with an overnight bag I brought the fear that I could pass a kidney stone at any time.

My greatest worry was being in a small coastal community where there was no hospital. In some places, the nearest healthcare facility was a three-hour drive away. This was also a concern expressed by the patient in the video. We worried that we would lose the freedom to travel; we would always have to carry prescription pain medication and check in advance if there was a medical facility within reasonable traveling distance.

My desire to be stone free (so that this would also be one less piece of "baggage" I would have to carry on visits to the coast) helped me cope with my anxiety over what I thought was going to be yet another painful procedure.

My first lithotripsy was a difficult experience. However, new advancements in the type of lithotripter used, as well as new medical techniques, had made lithotripsy more bearable. Also, I was a "new" second-time-around patient because I asked lots of questions. I was amazed at the difference in myself. Knowing what to expect and having some knowledge of the procedure left me less anxious during the second lithotripsy.

At the first lithotripsy, the urologist wanted me to have a stent, a thin, soft plastic tubing running from my kidney to my bladder to allow for safe passage of the shattered stone fragments, and to serve as an X-ray landmark; a spinal for anesthesia (done the night prior to the lithotripsy); and a catheter, along with a three-day hospitalization. While these medical procedures were not life threatening to my survival, they made life more uncomfortable and at times almost more painful than passing the kidney stone.

Along with a rather large stone, for the second lithotripsy, I brought a lot of "bad memories" from the first lithotripsy. I was scared by the first experience. No, that is not the word. I was petrified.

After expressing my concerns to my new urologist, and telling him I was an anxious patient, he felt it would be best for me to be given general anesthesia to put me to sleep. He explained that it was crucial not to move during the procedure and that if I did move I could add another 30 minutes to the surgery. Anesthesia also helps reduce respiratory and body movement.

I understood that quite well, and I liked the idea of sleeping through any discomfort. Not needing spinal anesthesia was also nice although it works well for many patients. However, I really wanted to remain awake. My goal was to be able to write about the procedure from a patient's point of view—and I couldn't do that if I let them put me to sleep.

After the visit with my urologist, I was given blood and urine tests at the out-patient surgery center. Then I completed a patient questionnaire for the staff anesthesiologist, filled out insurance forms, and signed hospital pre-admission forms in the unlikely event they might be necessary. Then I was told to relax!

I remember a story I heard years ago—most likely over the years it has turned into a fractured fairy tale. In the story, Alice in Wonderland is crying. The Queen asked Alice why she is crying.

"I am crying now so that when the time comes, I will not have anything to cry about," she said.

That is how I view any procedure done to my own body. I do a lot of crying before the actual experience so I can appear to be very brave.

> Fortunately, kidney stones are seldom life-threatening, although they can temporarily take the joy out of existence.
>
> **Allen J. Sheinman**
> **The Good News on Stones**
> **New Choices**
> **August 1989**

I arrived at the surgery center the following day at 8:00 a.m. for a 10:00 a.m. lithotripsy. I had had nothing to eat since midnight, and for the first time in my life involving any surgical procedure, I felt quite relaxed. This amazed me.

My doctor had arranged for the surgical nurse to administer a mild tranquilizer, and I was glad to receive it. I wanted to continue feeling tranquil. I sensed the fears of other patients undergoing surgical procedures. While I certainly had empathy for them, I needed to focus on myself and remain calm. A friend stayed with me during the two hours that I waited. Having someone to talk with helped me a lot. The nurses were helpful and answered all my questions.

The second-time-around lithotripsy did not require a catheter inserted into my bladder. I was extremely thankful and delighted about that. Also, my urologist told me I most likely would not require a stent. Just knowing that helped ease most of my fear.

Finally, it was my turn to travel on the gurney to the litho–tripter. Two friendly nurses from the surgical center guided my gurney down the long hallway to where the mobile kidney stone unit was "parked" out behind the surgery center. For a few brief seconds, I felt the warm summer sun on my face.

The gurney was placed on a lift. While it was far from an amusement park ride, I wondered if many patients felt they, too, were on a carnival ride. I am positive the effects of the tranquilizer had put a smile on my face as I contemplated this thought.

At the touch of a button, the mobile unit elevator lifted the gurney into what looked like a warehouse site! The entire side of the van seemed to open like an automatic garage door! Inside the unit it looked like a friendly neighbor's living room. It was nicely decorated with soothing wallpaper. There were two landscape paintings of the Pacific coast. This helped me to focus my thoughts on places I loved.

The anesthesiologist played an important role during the lithotripsy, serving as a communicator between the patient, and the physician. I found it was extremely important to communicate to him my concerns and exactly how I was feeling.

Looking back on my first lithotripsy, I felt uncomfortable because I did not communicate my feelings to the anesthesiologist. I felt that I was alone. I was a docile patient.

It was amazing the positive changes that took place when I voiced my opinions as a patient with my second lithotripsy! I was a new person the second time around—one who knew what to expect and one who wasn't afraid to ask questions. And this time I got the high quality of care I had expected the first time.

A whole new world of options opened up as soon as I moved onto the dry table of the lithotripter. I was again asked if I wanted general anesthesia or if I wanted to remain awake and receive medication as needed.

The anesthesiologist explained that if any part of the procedure was uncomfortable, I could safely be put to sleep within a minute. Having to make a last minute decision, especially under the effects of a mild tranquilizer, left me feeling uncertain.

I told the anesthesiologist that I had no idea what I wanted. This was the only frustrating part of the entire procedure.

With some of the newer lithotripter machines, only a local anesthetic is needed. I was fortunate to have one of the newest models on the market. The staff made the decision regarding anesthesia for me; I would receive pain medication as needed to see how well I could tolerate the procedure. The anesthesiologist explained this decision to my physician, who was surprised—especially after I had spent considerable time explaining how anxious I was.

The procedure began.

Within seconds, X-ray devices within the lithotripter located the first of five stones in my right kidney. I could feel the gentle nudging of the machine as it positioned my right side into the optimal position. I had been told not to move—not even to scratch my nose! As it turned out, I was able to maintain that exact position during the entire 1 and 1/2 hour-long procedure.

The urologist focused his greatest concern on the two largest of the five stones. One measured 15 mm in diameter (as large as the "O" in the the word "Stone" on this book's cover). Both were too large to pass through the ureter without some kind of assistance.

With lithotripsy, neither soft tissues nor bones are hurt by the thousands of shock waves. The brittle stone, however, absorbs the shock wave energy and shatters under the impact, breaking into sand-like particles that are easier to pass in the urine.

During the entire procedure, a loud noise below me resounded through the treatment room. The noise came from the lithotripter. As the procedure continued, the intensity of the shock waves could be felt, but was easily managed with pain medication. Two shock waves per second helped the stones crumble.

Typically, the stone begins to crumble after 200 to 400 shock waves. X-rays are used to determine what effect the shock waves are having on the stone. Hardly ten minutes had passed before the lithotripsy technician, who assisted my urologist, walked over and held my hand. "Your stone has taken on a new form already, Gail," he said. "It's no longer in one piece." I thought it would take a lot longer to break up the largest stone!

I told the anesthesiologist as soon as I felt the need for more pain medication. Within seconds, I could feel the medication's effect, and the procedure became easily tolerable. I was amazed at how well it was going.

An hour and a half later, at the end of the procedure, I had received over 10,000 shock waves. Six thousand shock waves were focused on one stone, and another 4,000 shock waves sent into the four smaller stones. Each shock wave carried a force of 5,000 to 15,000 pounds pressure per square inch. The force of a single shock wave has been likened to a "hearty slap on the back." The maximum number of shocks will vary depending on the location of the stone and the specific type of ESWL machine.

Finally, there was silence in the room. I could hear the lithotripter being shut off. Perhaps the silence was also there because of my obvious relief that it was over!

I slid once again back onto the gurney, and I was wheeled back out into the hot sun. My urologist walked alongside my gurney along with the two surgical nurses who had assisted during the procedure and the technician. He said that after lithotripsy, patients should be given sunglasses. But I was more than glad to see the sun!

But then again it was not quite over. Now it was important that I pass the stones by drinking large amounts of water. My doctor advised me to drink lots of fluids to maintain a strong urinary flow and help eliminate the stone fragments. I used a urine strainer that the surgery center gave me to recover the stone fragments.

Because I was not given general anesthesia, I was able to sit up in a chair in the recovery room. However, I could not stop my body from shaking. Some of the nurses felt that my body was responding to the utter relief I felt now that the procedure was finally over. The anesthesiologist felt that perhaps my blood sugar level was low since I had not eaten in over twelve hours.

Within minutes, I drank three small cans of apple juice and this helped me immensely. The shaking was subsiding.

I asked to use the bathroom. Even though I was still connected to an IV unit, it felt wonderful to be able to get up and walk. A recovery room nurse walked with me and stayed while I used the toilet being careful to strain all the urine. I was not prepared for the large amount of blood. I flushed the toilet. Heading off my panic, the recovery room nurse told me that this was very normal and that the bleeding would subside within 24 to 48 hours.

It actually took less time in my case; within 12 hours my urine appeared to be normal. (Following lithotripsy, the patient should expect the urine to have a pink or red discoloration for the first few days after treatment).

The nurse explained the small four-inch diameter, reddish patch over my right kidney was a reaction to the lithotripsy. (Some patients may find a small bruise). Although I was advised to call my physician if the bruise got larger, in actuality it got smaller and disappeared over the next four days.

The only discomfort I felt after lithotripsy was soreness over the right kidney. This was easily managed with pain medication. I was too sore to sleep on my right side, but after a week this also subsided.

I passed the majority of the larger stone fragments by the fifth day. An X-ray examination two weeks following lithotripsy showed that I had no stones.

This was remarkable and certainly not the case of most patients following lithotripsy. The standard regarding elimination of stone fragments following lithotripsy is that it may take up to three months. (Many patients contact me, worried, that after two weeks they still have stone fragments. Patients need to continue drinking large amounts of water and other beverages and remain as active as possible).

Some patients may experience pain, fever or nausea during the first three months. Such symptoms are of short duration and are treated with mild pain medication such as Tylenol or Motrin.

Though lithotripsy is a relatively painless procedure, it is considered a physically taxing treatment. I was amazed how tired I was for a few days afterwards. A friend stayed with me and took over all household responsibilities, including cooking. This helped me immensely. And while I love my children dearly, they went to visit their father for a short while. Several days of quiet, restful recovery without the responsibility of caring for others proved beneficial.

While there was some discomfort overall, I have to say that compared to a long hospital stay, a large scar from kidney surgery and weeks of recovery at home, lithotripsy helped me get back to living life again without the fear and pain of passing a kidney stone in the middle of the night.

Incredibly, a small stone fragment still remains to this day in my right kidney. I have been able to keep that stone fragment from growing larger, and it does not give me any pain at all—well, psychologically yes, but no physical pain. One problem with lithotripsy is that there is no guarantee that all stone fragments can be shattered small enough to pass.

I eventually had a third lithotripsy and again, did not pass all the stone fragments. This lithotripsy was performed a few days before New Year's Eve and in the midst of a major thunderstorm and flooding in California. The staff had to wrap me in large plastic sheeting so I wouldn't get soaked on the gurney to the lithotripsy van in the parking lot.

"Well, this is just fine," I said to myself. "I hope no other patient sees me this way because I must look quite dead wrapped in gray plastic material normally used for garbage bags."

This third procedure also did not require a stent, catheterization, or anesthesia. Performed by my second urologist, but at a different surgery center, I again encountered a major problem.

The anesthesiologist at this surgery center did not call me the previous night, and I found her attitude towards me condescending. Whenever I asked a question, she laughed it off. She never answered any of my questions! When I inquired about a tranquilizer prior to the procedure, she told me not to worry and that they would take care of it. I never received the tranquilizer. Since this had been previously discussed with my urologist, I could not believe her callous attitude.

A few weeks later I called her office and explained my absolute frustration with this anesthesiologist. Most doctors take these complaints seriously and want to hear your opinion. If you are still not satisfied, put your complaint in writing and send it to the Better Business Bureau, the State Medical Licensing Board, the local county medical society and the hospital or surgery center where the procedure was performed.

Looking toward the future, lithotripsy will continue to be the main surgical treatment for most kidney stones. Newer machines make the procedure more tolerable, but the key is understanding what is going on and reviewing the details with your urologist.

Some patients will need stents, special imaging techniques or repeat lithotripsy for difficult stones. A good urologist will explain his reasoning and technique as well and answer your questions.

CHAPTER EIGHTEEN

Stone Treatment by Surgery
Baskets, Lasers, Stents and Parachutes

Without a doubt, the best way to get rid of a kidney stone is to allow it to pass spontaneously so there is no risk of surgical misadventures, complications or anesthesia-related problems. Fortunately, most stones will eventually pass by themselves, usually painlessly and often without the patient even aware of it. That is why doctors ask patients with stones to carefully strain all their urine in case a stone is passed. The one time a patient forgets to strain the urine is probably when the stone will pass and the opportunity to collect it for analysis is gone forever!

If the stone is 4 mm or less, then there is a 90 percent chance of spontaneous passage. Stones 5 mm (about 1/4 inch) to 7 mm in size have a 50 percent chance of passing, while stones larger than 7 mm only rarely pass by themselves.

Urologists and the Decision to Perform Surgery

Urologists are surgeons who specialize in treating diseases of the urinary tract, especially where surgery might be necessary. Urologists generally give stones every possible chance to pass by themselves before any surgery is considered. If there is no compelling reason to recommend surgery, urologists will often wait several months for a small stone in the ureter to pass before recommending any surgery. If a small ureteral stone has not moved in about three months, it probably is not going to pass by itself and surgery should probably be considered. Previous stone surgeries or infections can make it harder for a subsequent stone to pass due to scar tissue causing a narrowing of the ureter. This scarring is called a stricture.

There are certain conditions and situations where we probably should not wait for a stone to pass. These conditions include:

- Severe kidney infection not responding to antibiotics
- Blockage in a solitary kidney
- Severe pain for more than 24 hours which cannot be adequately controlled by medication
- Stone in a transplanted kidney
- Anatomical abnormality of the urinary system
- Stone too large to pass (generally 8 mm or more in diameter)
- Staghorn or Struvite (Infection) stones
- Kidney or renal failure
- Scar tissue or strictures which narrow the ureters
- Multiple stones

The decision to perform a surgery and the nature of the intervention should be discussed in detail with a urologist. You can and should talk to your regular physician, but it is the urologist who is the real specialist in getting rid of your stone.

How to Find the Most Qualified Urologist

When possible, ask for a urologist who is Board Certified. This means that the urologist has received at least five years of specialized training in urological surgery and has passed several tough examinations given by the American Board of Urology. Many excellent urologists are not Board Certified because they have not been in practice long enough to take all the examinations or for other good reasons. Don't be afraid to ask about your urologist's training and experience. An affiliation or clinical faculty appointment at a medical school or university hospital is desirable but not mandatory. Ask your regular physician to recommend someone he would use himself. Your local or state medical associations will also be able to give you quality information.

Often, the nurses who work in the hospital will have strong opinions about the qualifications and expertise of the urologists who work there. You can also contact the American Urological Association at (410) 727-1100 who will supply you with the names and addresses of its members, all of whom must be Board Certified as a condition of membership.

The Kidney Stone Network also maintains a Physician Referral to stone prevention specialists. They can be contacted at 1-800-2-KIDNEYS.

The urologist should take the time to answer all your questions, review the nature and type of procedure along with possible alternatives, complications and side effects. Remember, you can always ask for a second opinion or another urologist!

Surgical Procedures for Stone Removal

There are several different types of surgical procedures that are available to remove, bypass or fragment urinary stones. Stone basket extractions, the use of stents, ureteroscopy, internal stone fragmenting devices, extracorporeal shock wave lithotripsy (ESWL), percutaneous removal techniques and traditional "open" surgery of the ureter and kidneys are reviewed in the following pages.

Stone Basket Extraction

When a stone is in the lower third of the ureter and below the level of the major leg blood vessels, it is often possible to grab the stone in a special basket and pull it out.

First, the patient is given an anesthetic to eliminate any pain or discomfort during the procedure. A special telescope is passed into the bladder and the opening into the ureter is identified. (This part of the procedure is called a cystoscopy). Often, a retrograde pyelogram is performed first. A small plastic tube is inserted through the telescope into the end of the ureter. Dye or contrast is gently injected for an X-ray picture of the entire ureter. Any blockages, kinks, stones or strictures will be visible on this X-ray.

Once the stone is located, one of three types of stone baskets will be selected. They all share a handle with an operating lever to open and close the basket and a long covered tube within which is the wire basket itself. When the basket is retracted within the small plastic sheath, the tube is small enough to pass into the ureter and hopefully reach or pass the stone. The handle is then operated and the basket is pushed out of the tube and into the ureter. The shape of the resulting basket is what is different between the three types of stone baskets. All of these baskets are used with fluroscopy and with special telescopes so that their orientation and activities can be monitored by the urologist. Stone baskets are named after the doctors who invented them.

"Dormia" or Spiral Basket

The "Dormia" or spiral basket is the oldest, traditional type of stone basket. It may have anywhere from three to eight wires in the form of a gentle spiral. In general, the fewer the wires in the basket, the larger the stone it can handle. A larger number of wires is better able to hold onto smaller stones and fragments. In operation, the basket is usually passed beyond the stone and gently pulled back while being slowly rotated. The intention is for the stone to fall within the central core of the open basket which can then be closed, trapping the stone inside. It can then be slowly pulled out of the ureter.

"Segura" or Flat Wire Basket

The "Segura" or flat wire basket is a newer type of stone basket designed by Dr. Joseph Segura, a respected urologist at the Mayo Clinic. It has four wires and they are arranged something like an orange cut into quarters. The wires themselves are flat which gives the basket considerable opening force to enlarge or dilate the ureter but it cannot be rotated without risking ureteral damage. This basket is usually used with a special telescope designed to pass into the ureter called a ureteroscope. The basket is opened next to the stone which has to pass between two of the wires. When a stone is inside the core, the basket can be closed and the stone removed.

"Leslie" Parachute Basket

The "Leslie" Parachute Basket has a truly unique design. Both of the other baskets are totally symmetrical with the top and bottom portions appearing to be exactly the same. The "Leslie" Parachute Basket is the only asymmetrical basket design available. When open, this basket has two wires on the

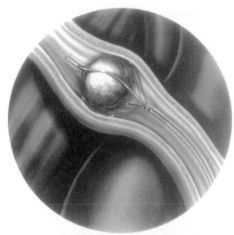

Segura Stone Basket® maximizes opening force and is most useful in "tight" quarters. The flat wire design provides added strength.

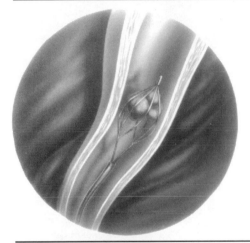

Leslie "Parachute" Basket® is uniquely adapted to the challenges of multiple stone retrieval and intracorporeal lithotripsy. The basket works like a small net by spreading apart multiple wires at the top of the basket. This is especially useful for smaller stones and fragments.

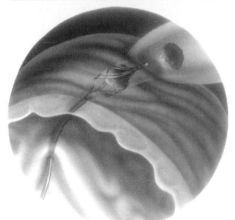

Gemini or Spiral-type Basket® was the first wire basket design and is still the most commonly used basket.

Illustrations courtesy of Boston Scientific/Microvasive

ILLUSTRATION A

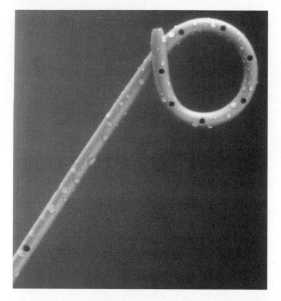

Double-J Stent® promotes excellent drainage while the pigtail shape prevents the stent from migrating out of place. The inside of the curl is approximately the size of a dime.

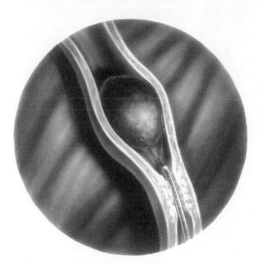

Forceps can grab and release stones easily, but holds stones less securely than the basket designs.

Illustrations courtesy of Boston Scientific/Microvasive

ILLUSTRATION B

bottom end which split up at the midpoint of the basket into a network or canopy of six to eight wires at the top. This design was intended to create a large opening in the bottom of the basket to allow stones to pass into the central core while still having multiple wires to act as a net to capture and hold any stones tight without letting them escape. The basket is opened above the stone and then gently pulled downwards. In practice, this technique works best on small and medium sized stones of 7 mm or less diameter and for multiple stones. It is also excellent when used like a net to capture the small stone fragments created when internal stone fragmentation devices are used. Different versions of the basket are under development with fewer, thicker wires to make it more effective with larger stones. (In case you were wondering, the "Leslie" Parachute Basket was designed by Dr. Stephen W. Leslie, a noted urologist who is also one of the co-authors of this book).

Some of the baskets are used with small balloon dilators to stretch and spread open the lower end of the ureter. This is the place where the ureter is most narrow, where it enters the bladder. In some cases, the captured stone is too large to be pulled out of the ureter even when tightly held in a stone basket. When this happens, urologists use an internal fragmentation instrument to break up the stone into smaller pieces or use a balloon dilator to gently stretch open the lowest end of the ureter to allow the stone and basket to pass out.

Ureteroscopy

This is a technique where the urologist uses a specially designed telescope to pass into the bladder and then up into the ureter. The telescope is longer and thinner than the one used to inspect only the bladder. There are two types of ureteroscopes: rigid and flexible.

Rigid ureteroscopes are the kind generally used in the lower third of the ureter for inspection and stone removal. Older scopes required balloon dilation of the lower end of the ureter, but some of the newer scopes are very small and tapered which allows them to pass in most people without dilation. The scope itself has several passageways which allow for irrigation, suction, and the passage of guidewires and specially designed baskets and graspers. Through these scopes, the urologist can use a variety of internal stone fragmenting devices like lasers to breakup the stones or better manipulate a basket to grasp and extract stones from the ureter.

Flexible ureteroscopes are used mainly to inspect the upper ureter and the inside of the kidney. The scope is made of fiberglass which can bend but still transmit a clear picture. Some stones in the upper ureter can still be fragmented using this instrument, but it is more difficult to operate and some of the internal fragmentation devices cannot be used with a flexible scope.

Internal Stone Fragmentation Devices

The development of telescopes that allow surgeons to actually look into the ureters and see stones made it possible to use various probes, baskets and graspers to remove the stones efficiently. Unfortunately, many stones are just too big to pull out easily and need to be broken up or fragmented first. Use of an instrument, machine or probe to fragment a stone is called lithotripsy.

The challenge in fragmenting a stone inside the body is how to deliver enough power or energy to break up a stone as hard as any pebble you might find outside on the sidewalk or by a riverbank, while not injuring the soft and delicate ureter that is right next to it.

Ultrasonic Lithotripsy

The first of these devices used high frequency sound waves, called ultrasound, that were delivered by a solid, rigid rod through a telescope in the bladder or ureter and directly into the stone being treated. This energy causes the probe to act like an engraver or drill and can break apart even the hardest stones. It does not injure the ureter because it only has full effect on hard objects, not the soft, fleshy walls of the ureter. This is much the same way an engraver works. You can touch the tip of the engraver and it just feels like it's buzzing. But when you touch it to something hard and firm, like a piece of wood, it etches a groove in that object. Newer forms of internal fragmentation devices have pretty much replaced the older ultrasound units, but they are still around and are still used occasionally.

Electrohydraulic Lithotripsy (EHL)

This machine is able to generate a small but powerful spark at the tip of a flexible probe. The probe is placed through a telescope very close to the stone, but not touching it. When the spark goes off, a strong shock wave is created. This shock wave is similar to the sonic boom of a supersonic aircraft. It causes intense vibrations inside the stone but passes harmlessly through the surrounding soft tissue. Essentially, it vibrates the stone until it crumbles. This is the same principal used in extracorporeal shock wave lithotripsy or ESWL except that the shock wave generator is miniaturized and placed next to the stone.

Electrohydraulic lithotripsy or EHL is a very powerful device for fragmenting stones. it can be used anywhere in the urinary system including the kidney. Since the probes are flexible, they can pass through either the rigid or flexible ureteroscopes. The machine itself is relatively inexpensive, so EHL has become a popular and widely used device for internal stone fragmentation.

Lasers

The "Holmium" laser can fragment and even vaporize some stones. The probes used are very thin but may not be very flexible which limits their use somewhat. The color of the laser light is such that the laser energy is absorbed by the stone but is reflected by blood and soft tissues like the ureter. This makes the laser very safe. Since the fiber is so thin and narrow, very small and delicate telescopes can be used. The fiber is placed in direct contact with the stone and the laser is fired.

Lasers are powerful enough to break up just about any type of stone. They are more effective than EHL, ultrasound or pneumatic devices like the Lithoclast described below. The "Holmium" laser can quickly break up stones that are difficult or impossible to fragment with other therapies. When available, the "Holmium" laser is currently the preferred surgical technique, along with ESWL described later, for internal stone fragmentation. The main problem with lasers is the very high cost of a laser generator.

Lithoclast

This is the strange name of a new device for internal fragmentation that has been used in Europe for several years but only recently became available in the United States. The

Lithoclast is actually a small pneumatic hammer designed for fragmentation of ureteral stones. The probe for the device is thin but solid and has only limited flexibility. At the base of the probe, there is a small pellet inside a closed chamber. This pellet is fired at the base of the probe by compressed air. When the pellet hits the base of the probe, all of the energy from the pellet is transmitted directly to the opposite tip of the probe and into the stone that it is touching. This is similar in principle to croquet where hitting a solid, stationary ball with a mallet transmits all the energy to the neighboring ball in contact with the first one. Anyway, this banging or hammering is repeated rapidly until the stone is shattered. The technique works quite well and is very safe. The machine itself is much less expensive than a laser and safer than the EHL.

Extracorporeal Shock Wave Lithotripsy (ESWL)

Extracorporeal shock wave lithotripsy or ESWL, which is pronounced "Ess-wall," is the revolutionary kidney stone fragmentation device that is commonly known as the "Stone Machine." It was originally developed in Germany and came to the United States in 1984. Since then, it has become the established standard for treating virtually all kidney stones except a few special cases.

The original machine used a large tub of warm water and a padded metal frame. The patient was fully anesthetized and placed on the frame which was then lowered into the water. At the bottom of the tank there is a large spark plug in a small open chamber. The walls of this chamber are carefully shaped to concentrate all of the shocks waves produced by the spark plug to a very small, specific point above the chamber. This area is identified by two fluoroscope machines that are at 90 degrees to each other and calibrated so that the maximum shock wave blast impact is identified as the exact center of the target areas on both scopes. Essentially, if both fluroscopes show a stone to be on target, then it will receive the full force of the shock waves being produced by the spark plug two feet below. The patient and frame are moved and adjusted so that any stones in

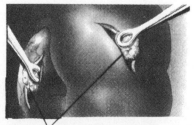

Surgical removal of stones from renal pelvis and kidney

Forceps   Basket   Electro-hydraulic   Laser

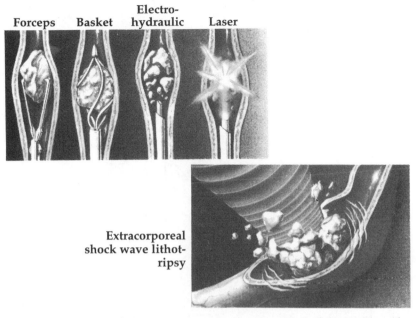

Extracorporeal shock wave lithotripsy

Illustrations courtesy of Blaine Company Inc., Pharmaceuticals, Erlanger, Kentucky.

the kidneys or ureters are located exactly at this focal point. When the spark plug is energized, it separates the water into oxygen and hydrogen which then immediately recombine to form water again. This reaction is so fast that it creates a very powerful shock wave which is directed to the focal point as explained earlier.

Shock waves pass harmlessly through the body and soft tissues. Only when they hit something hard and rigid, like a stone, will they cause any fragmentation. Actually, the stones tend to crumble much like you would crumble a sugar cube between your fingers. It's like they are vibrated to pieces.

While ESWL appears to be harmless, you can expect some blood in the urine for a few days after the procedure. Small stone fragments will begin to pass and should be collected for analysis. Even very tiny fragments like sand or gravel can reveal important information when properly analyzed.

If you could step up into an original ESWL suite which was operating, you would see a brief flash of light, much like a flash bulb, and hear a loud clap. This would be repeated every few seconds until the entire ESWL treatment was finished. Usually between 1,500 and 3,000 shocks, each done one at a

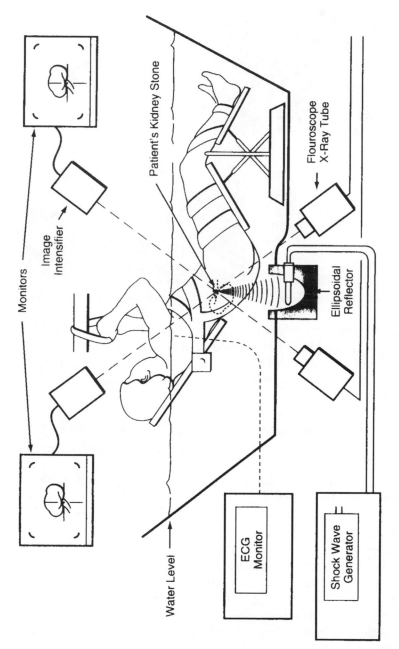

First-Generation Extracorporeal Shock Wave Lithotriptor
Illustration courtesy of Blaine Company Inc., Pharmaceuticals, Erlanger, Kentucky.

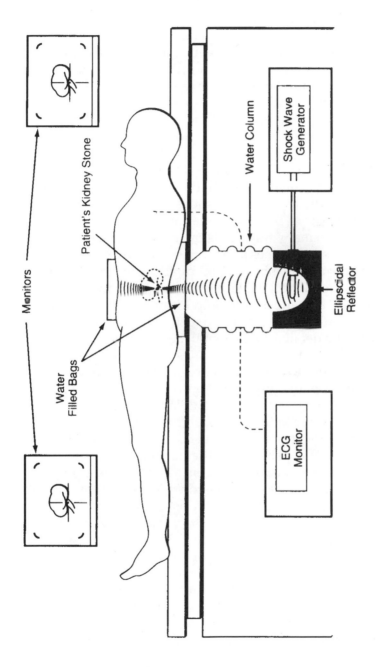

Second-Generation Extracorporeal Shock Wave Lithotriptor
Illustration courtesy of Blaine Company Inc., Pharmaceuticals, Erlanger, Kentucky.

time, are needed for each stone that is being treated depending on the hardness of the stone and its location.

Newer generations of these ESWL machines may require more shocks but need less anesthesia and have done away with the tub of water. Some use crystals that vibrate when electrified to create the shock wave, but many still use some type of spark plug encased in a water filled drum which is placed in contact with the patient. It works quite well and the patient doesn't get wet! Still, many urologists prefer to use the original water tub machine, called the HM-3, because it delivers the most powerful shock waves and can break up harder stones.

Stones anywhere in the urinary system can be fragmented using the ESWL machine. Stones in the ureter can be difficult to see and generally require more shock treatments than stones located in the kidneys. Stents are often used to help avoid clogging from too many fragments trying to pass at once, and to help identify small stones and stones in the ureters. (Stents are thin, hollow plastic tubes placed by the urologist prior to ESWL. They extend from the kidney through the ureter to the urinary bladder and are used to help locate hard to see stones and help drain the kidneys. See the section on stents which follows for more details). Occasionally, even the stents are insufficient help in finding some stones, especially those that don't contain any calcium such as uric acid stones. In these cases, a slender, hollow tube called a ureteral catheter is placed through a telescope just prior to the ESWL. This tube extends from the center of the kidney, through the ureter and bladder, and out the urethra. It can then be used to inject contrast directly into the renal pelvis from the outside during the ESWL treatment. This allows excellent visualization of the central part of the kidney and any stones located there.

There is considerable controversy as to whether ureteroscopy or ESWL is better for stones in the lower ureter. Both techniques work quite well, but ESWL requires less anesthesia and is less invasive. However, if the urologist is very skilled in ureteroscopy, he may recommend that technique first. Talk to the urologist about the alternatives and the relative pros and cons of your particular situation.

Only very large stones over one inch in diameter and branched or staghorn stones should not be fragmented with ESWL alone. In these cases, a combined approach called

"Sandwich Therapy" using both ESWL and percutaneous procedures, described below, are preferred.

ESWL is one of the few kidney stone treatment modalities than can be safely used in children. It is not recommended, however, during pregnancy.

Percutaneous Procedures

Percutaneous literally means "through the skin." The technique requires making a small hole in the body on the side where the stone or obstruction is located. Local anesthetic is used to numb the skin first. Using X-ray or ultrasound imaging, a needle is passed through the skin and into the central collection part of the kidney called the renal pelvis. A guidewire is passed through the needle and into the kidney. The needle is removed and the passageway is dilated or stretched using a series of plastic dilators or a specially designed balloon. This enlarges the passage until it is big enough to allow passage of either an operating telescope, graspers, stone baskets or internal stone fragmenting probes. Because a hole or opening is made into the kidney, this technique is considered more invasive than any of the other procedures already described. There is the risk that the probes or needles may injure a major blood vessel in the kidney and require further surgery. Nevertheless, this is an excellent method for removing large, branched stones called staghorns. Since this type of stone is relatively rare, even many urologists have limited experience with percutaneous surgical procedures. If your urologist recommends this type of surgery, make sure you ask him his experience and success rate with this particular method.

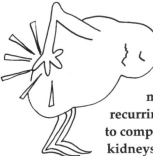

People with stones would sometimes lose their kidneys before the invention of modern non-invasive treatments and preventive therapies. The multiple operations needed to remove recurring stones often left scar tissue which lead to complications. Eventually, some patients' kidneys stopped functioning altogether.

Open or Traditional Surgery

Open surgery refers to the traditional type of surgery which used to be done quite often for stones. The patient is place on an operating table and an incision is made in the lower abdomen, mid-abdomen or flank depending on where the stone is located. When the kidney or ureter is reached, a small incision is made and the stones removed. The incisions are closed with stitches and the patient is returned to his room.

Recovery from these surgeries usually takes weeks and there is considerable pain. Scar tissue can develop and cause more stones to be created in the future as well as strictures that will block the passage of urine and any new stones. We try to avoid open surgery whenever possible and it is seldom done anymore for kidney stones. Only in exceptional cases will open surgery still be required for any type of stone disease. Fortunately, it has pretty much been retired and replaced with the more advanced surgical techniques previously described.

Stents

Many patients complain about stents. Amy writes that she "had shock wave lithotripsy (one week ago) and was left with a stent in her body which was extremely painful and uncomfortable. It has taken me a week to feel okay. The doctor told me that I still have two kidney stones and may have to do this lithotripsy again. I do not want to have it because I won't be able to tolerate the stent. "

As a patient, I also felt traumatized by the stent. I insisted that it be removed a few days following lithotripsy. But stents are important, often essential and occasionally life-saving for some patients.

What is this demon that so many stone patients fear? A stent is a thin, slender, hollow plastic tube of variable length that is used to permit drainage and bypass obstructions, slow the passage of stone fragments after ESWL and stabilize or support the ureter after various types of surgeries. It is sometimes used to help identify the ureters when complex pelvic cancer operations are performed.

The length of the stent is between 20 and 30 cm which is essentially the length of the ureter. They are available in 2 cm increments. Each stent is made of a plastic and/or silicone composite and has a series of small holes throughout its length to help with drainage. The material of the stent has a "memory" which allows each end of the stent to return to a gentle curl whenever it is released. (These curls are sometimes called pigtails which they resemble and that's why stents are sometimes called double pigtails or double-J's). The curls' job is to keep the stent in place until they are removed. One curl should be in the urinary bladder while the other should coil up just inside the kidney.

Stents are placed through special telescopes in the bladder while their position is checked by X-ray and fluroscopy. A guidewire is placed first and then the stent is pushed over the wire into the ureter. The wire is easier to position and it straightens out the curls of the stent during placement.

Stents generally come in three widths: 6 French, 7 French and 8.5 French. (French means the circumference in mm). It's a good idea to ask the urologist for the length and French size of the stent used. If you ever need another stent for any reason, it is helpful to know the size that worked once before.

Stents are used to bypass stones that can't be moved or extracted for some reason. This procedure relieves the pain from the blockage even if it doesn't actually remove the stone. This is often a useful technique in pregnant women or in patients who are too ill to have any more definitive therapy performed at that time. Leaving a stent in place will gently dilate or stretch the ureter. This may allow the stone to move or pass easier once the stent is removed and can also be used to treat strictures or scarred, narrowed portions of the ureter. Stents can also help relieve the pain after balloon dilation of the lower ureter which would otherwise develop painful spasms.

During ESWL procedures, it is often difficult to find some of the smaller stones, especially if they are in the ureter. Stents permit the ESWL to better pinpoint the stones for fragmentation. The stent acts as a landmark that is easy to see on the fluoroscopes of the ESWL machine. The stent will also slow the passage of stone fragments when large stones are treated to prevent clogging.

Large stones usually require stents to be placed before ESWL to prevent clogging of the ureter from too many fragments trying to pass all at once. Blockage of the ureter from a column of stone fragments after ESWL is called "Steinstrasse" which is German for "Street of Stones." The Germans who developed the first ESWL machines didn't use stents at first and they had these types of problems especially when the original stones were 10 mm or larger in size. This is similar to dumping a 10 pound bag of flour into your sink all at once. Chances are the sink will clog from too much flour at one time. If you use a teaspoon to slowly empty the bag of flour a little at a time, you will be able to empty the bag without clogging the sink. This is exactly how a stent is supposed to help avoid the problem: by forcing the abundant stone fragments to take turns passing alongside the stent while maintaining adequate drainage of the kidney through the stent's open central channel. Steinstrasse is usually treated with simple observation if there are no symptoms or any infections. Sixty-five percent will eventually resolve spontaneously. If further intervention is necessary, this may include either more ESWL, ureteroscopy or percutaneous drainage of the kidney through an external tube placed in the flank.

Stents usually don't bother most people very much, but there are always exceptions. Be sure to discuss the pros and cons with your urologist. If there is a good reason for placing a stent, you should probably accept it. If it proves to be too uncomfortable, it can be easily removed in the urologist's office.

Most stents come with strings attached. A thin thread is sewn onto the end of the stent. The thread is used by the urologist during surgery to help move the stent into proper position. Usually the thread is removed just after the stent is placed. Occasionally, this thread will be left dangling out of the bladder where it can be used to remove the stent at a later date. If you have a stent with such a thread left hanging out of the bladder, be sure that you don't accidentally pull on it or you could move the stent out of position or even remove it prematurely.

Stone Free-Now What?

The procedure is over and finally, at long last, one is stone free. Chances are greater than one in two that the patient will suffer another stone within five to ten years if there is no prevention program.

CHAPTER NINETEEN

Nutrition: What You Eat May Lead You Down the Rocky Road of Life

B enjamin Franklin is said to have stood on his head while eating blackberry jelly in an attempt to dislodge a stone in his bladder!

While he may have been helping gravity dislodge stones by standing on his head, it's a different story for that blackberry jelly. The blackberry jelly may have contributed to further stone formation.

Today, we sometimes forget that patients with kidney stones can benefit from less glamorous therapies—like diet therapy. Many experts believe that nutrition can help prevent stone recurrence.

> Food was becoming my "enemy." The foods I loved best seemed to be the ones contributing most to those painful stones.
>
> —Gail Savitz

Sweet potatoes and spinach, two of the few vegetables I really like, were now "restricted" because of their oxalate content! A cup of sweet potatoes (boiled and mashed) provided a hefty dose of 184 mg of oxalate while one cup of frozen, boiled spinach added another 1,230 mg of oxalate. Chocolate was also high in oxalate. One ounce jolted my kidneys another 33 mg. And to think I'd have to forego one of life's greatest pleasures! I drank gallons of Indian iced tea in the summer, unaware that each cup added another 185 mg punch of oxalate.

Doctors often recommend changing eating habits to prevent recurrences, whether or not drugs are prescribed.

Over time I learned that the objective should be to limit excesses rather than curb intake completely. Using the I.R.S. Plan (see Chapter 15) and drinking more water on those occasions when I do have sweet potatoes has helped me prevent new stones.

While eating certain foods can increase mineral concentrations, I've found few patients are given detailed lists of foods to avoid.

> Only 22 U.S. medical schools required a course on nutrition in 1989-1990. About 100 schools offered an elective course in nutrition, but only 5% of medical students took that elective according to a report in the *American Journal of Clinical Nutrition*.
>
> **University of California at Berkeley**
> ***Wellness Letter*, March 1992**

A Highly Recommended Resource

There are many books suggested as recommended reading throughout this book. However, one book in particular should absolutely be purchased by all kidney stone formers, especially those with oxalate-containing stones. The General Clinical Research Center of the University of California San Diego Medical Center has published "Oxalate Content of Selected Foods—with Recipes and Menu Suggestions." This wonderful spiral-bound $12 book provides the most complete selection of foods by both food groups and name brands and contains the oxalate values for a wide variety of foods.

The oxalate content of a food may vary depending on soil conditions, time of harvest and processing. In addition, differences in the various ways foods are analyzed can add to the complexity of determining an absolute value for a food. Normal dietary intake of oxalate averages about 100 to 120 mg per day. In healthy people, much of the dietary oxalate is not absorbed. It forms an insoluble calcium salt in the small intestine and is excreted in the stool.

Low oxalate recipes are provided for French Toast Bake, salads and side dishes including California Wild Rice and several entrees.

One of the most fascinating facts from the oxalate book is that Coca-Cola® contains trace amounts of oxalate, a fact suggested by many other researchers throughout the world. Teas are listed by brand name (and some are quite shocking as to oxalate content).

Information on ordering the book can be found on page 269 in the Resources Chapter of this book.

Nutrients That Prevent Stone Formation

Nutrients which have been associated with calcium stone disease are oxalate, protein, and sodium as well as alcohol and some fluids like tea or cola-flavored beverages. Years ago it was believed dietary calcium contributed to kidney stones but as previously mentioned in this book, it has been found that a lack of dietary calcium can increase stone formation. The landmark study by Gary Curhan, M.D. of Harvard also revealed that:

- The quarter of men with the highest calcium consumption had a 34 percent lower risk of stones than did the quarter with the lowest intake.

- Men with the highest consumption of potassium, which is contained in fruits and vegetables, had only half the risk of developing kidney stones.

- A high fluid intake was associated with a 29 percent lower risk.

Why calcium might be good rather than bad is hard to explain.

Foods high in oxalate increase the risk of stones, but calcium blocks oxalate absorption from the intestinal tract.

Dr. Curhan recommends that people worried about stones make sure they get the recommended daily allowance of calcium (about 800 milligrams for most adults). This is the equivalent of just over three 8-ounce glasses of milk. The recommended amount for pregnant and nursing women is 1,200 milligrams.

The Calcium Information Center (1-800-321-2681) advises patients with kidney stones to contact their health care provider before beginning supplemental calcium.

New York Hospital-Cornell Medical Center and **Oregon Health Sciences University** operate a toll-free telephone number that provides recorded information about calcium intake. The number is (800) 321-2681. Leave your name, address, phone number and question. You can expect a response back in about a week.

Or write to:
The Calcium Information Center,
New York Hospital-Cornell Medical Center,
515 East 71st St., S-904, New York, NY 10021.

They offer several free, excellent publications on calcium.

The National Center for Nutrition and Dietetics can provide answers to diet and nutritional questions by mail or telephone. Call: (312) 899- 4853.

Or write to:
National Center for Nutrition and Dietetics,
American Dietetic Association,
216 West Jackson Blvd., Suite 800, Chicago, IL 60606-6995

According to a medical report by Fredric L. Coe, M.D., Joan H. Parks, M.B.A., and John R. Asplin, M.D., published in *The New England Journal of Medicine,* a simple dietary excess of oxalate increases urinary oxalate up to 50 to 60 mg daily (normal urinary oxalate is less than 40 mg per day). Specifically, foods such as spinach, rhubarb, Swiss chard, cocoa, beets, peppers, wheat germ, pecans, peanuts, okra, chocolate and lime peel are all suspect.

Treatment for patients with excessively high urinary oxalate includes altering the diet to avoid excess oxalate. Patients should make follow-up visits so their physicians can test their urine and blood.

A moderate dietary calcium restriction of 800 mg/day is often helpful in reducing excessive urinary calcium levels particularly if due to intestinal calcium hyperabsorption. This corresponds to roughly one or two servings of dairy products per day.

However, patients with Renal Calcium Leak and even some with intestinal calcium hyperabsorption will not respond to dietary calcium restrictions and could develop a negative calcium balance. Some people will be unable or unwilling to follow dietary restrictions. For these reasons, follow-up urinary calcium studies are essential.

Severe dietary calcium restrictions should be avoided because of the risk of increased free oxalate absorption. This is caused by the lack of dietary calcium which would otherwise bind to the intestinal oxalate, preventing its absorption. Moderation of excessive dietary oxalate should always accompany any calcium intake restrictions to avoid increasing urinary oxalate levels. Pregnant women, children and those at high risk for osteoporosis should be particularly careful to avoid any severe dietary calcium restrictions.

Good Food Sources for Calcium

Calcium is the most abundant mineral in the human body. Of the two to three pounds of calcium in the average body, 99 percent is stored in the bones and teeth. The remaining one percent plays a crucial role in muscle contraction, blood clotting, regulation of blood pressure, nerve transmission and other body processes.

Good food sources for calcium include 1 cup milk, low- fat or skim (300 mg.), 1 cup yogurt (300 mg.), two 1-ounce slices reduced fat cheese (300 mg.), 2 Tbs. blackstrap molasses, (284 mg.), 11 dried figs, 269 mg., 1 cup cooked white beans (81 mg.), 1 cup cottage cheese (204 mg.) and 1/2 cup ice cream (88 mg.). Keep in mind that caffeine, salty snacks, some soft drinks, alcohol, smoking and too much protein all speed up calcium loss.

What About Vegetarians?

As stated previously, a diet high in animal protein is linked to increased stone formation. This may be why the number of Americans who are stone prone is increasing. However, vegetarians and their friends are not necessarily becoming stone-free.

We seem to have a mismatch between the evolutionary design of our kidneys and the functional burden we place on them by our modern eating habits. The average meat-eating

American consumes 100 grams of protein per day, two to three times the Recommended Dietary Allowance, with most of the protein coming from animal products.

Vegetarians are also at risk for kidney stones if they eat a high oxalate diet from fruits and vegetables. For example, raw, firm tofu is a moderate oxalate source and depending on the amount eaten can greatly contribute to stone formation.

Some of the same non-dairy calcium-rich foods are high sources of oxalate. These include spinach, collards, kale, turnip greens, okra, asparagus, baby lima beans, artichokes and tofu.

Will Wine Make You Whine?

The role alcoholic beverages play in diet can be significant. Both wine and spirits can impair the ability of kidneys to eliminate uric acid from the blood. Thus, patients who have restricted their diet due to uric acid must be prudent with their use of alcohol; some are advised to eliminate it entirely, at least until appropriate uric acid-lowering drugs have had a chance to work.

Studies performed on beverages show that 12 fluid ounces of Stout, Guiness Draft, Lager, Tuborg and Pilsner beer is considered a high oxalate food source. And if you thought your Budweiser (12 fluid ounces) would help flush out stone-prone kidneys, well think again. That "Bud" is considered a moderate oxalate beverage. Unspecified draft beer is also a moderate source of oxalate.

Tests performed on red, rose and white wine show those beverages contain little or no oxalate.

Kidney Stones: The Disease of Affluence

Diet is believed to be a major contributor to the high rate of kidney stones in affluent countries. Researchers have found that "renal stone formers could be predisposed to stones because of their dietary patterns." Some research suggests that a 'rich' diet makes men more prone to calcium stones than women, whereas metabolic abnormalities play a more prominent role in stone formation in women.

A Japanese study revealed that kidney stone disease there has tripled since World War II, a change linked to the westernization of the Japanese diet. In a previous study, researchers from Kinki University in Osaka found that men with kidney stone disease ate more protein and less calcium than did healthy men, and often ate large, late dinners with short intervals between dinner and retiring. The researchers believe that "individual dietary management should be the primary measure" for preventing kidney stone disease at least in Japan.

Dietary Fiber, Rice Bran

Adding fiber to one's diet has been shown to decrease the urinary calcium and oxalate levels.

Researchers have also discovered that defatted rice bran (which contains phytin) binds calcium in the intestine and decreases urinary calcium output. This may prevent calcium stones from recurring in patients with high urinary calcium. The study followed 49 patients who received rice bran for more than three years. The results showed an obvious decline in stone formation rate, as compared with the three years immediately preceding treatment. In 30 patients (61.2 percent), no new stones formed during rice bran treatment.

The authors suggest that, while rice bran therapy is effective in reducing the recurrence of calcium stones, combining it with other preventive measures may be necessary for continued effectiveness.

Vitamin B-6 and Magnesium

Alan Wasserstein, M.D., director of the Stone Evaluation Center at the Hospital of the University of Pennsylvania advises his patients to take vitamin B-6 and magnesium supplements because he feels they tend to reduce oxalate levels and inhibit stone formation.

Canadian researchers report similar results with these vitamin supplements. It's important to know that some drugs can reduce magnesium levels (digitalis and oral diuretics).

Good food sources of magnesium include leafy, green vegetables (eaten raw), nuts (especially almonds and cashews), soybeans, seeds and whole grains. However, most of these foods are also high in oxalate!

> "As I see it, except for these supplements (250 to 500 milligrams of magnesium and 10 to 20 milligrams of vitamin B6), nothing more is needed either to prevent or dissolve kidney or bladder stones than a diet that furnishes adequate amounts of every nutrient including calcium."
>
> Adelle Davis
> *Let's Get Well*

Dietary Purines (High Stone Risk Proteins)

Urinary uric acid is primarily a result of the metabolic breakdown of body proteins and dietary protein (purine) intake. Excess dietary purines are the main cause of the high urinary uric acid levels often associated with calcium oxalate kidney stone disease. The relatively few patients who have high urinary uric acid levels from medical or liver disorders causing increased uric acid production by the body itself will probably be unresponsive to control by dietary measures alone.

The foods highest in purines include all meats, especially organ meats, poultry, seafood and beans. A restriction of 2 to 4 ounces of meat a day is recommended. Should dietary purine restriction alone be unsuccessful, additional treatment with allopurinol may be needed.

Dietary Acid Ash

High acid ash diets should be avoided in patients with low urinary citrate levels and those with very acid urines. The high acid ash will also contribute to uric acid stone disease and tends to increase the risk of calcium stones associated with elevated uric acid levels. Dietary acid ash content usually corresponds to animal protein intake (meat, poultry and fish). Other high acid ash foods include bread, crackers, cream soups, cranberries, plums, prunes, corn, lentils, noodles, rice, pastries, popcorn and most nuts. A high acid ash diet will tend to increase urinary acid, reduce citrate excretion, increase urinary calcium and increase urinary uric acid. These changes increase the risk of formation of both calcium and uric acid stones. Population studies clearly demonstrate a correlation between dietary animal protein and kidney stone formation.

Urinary sulfate level is a useful indicator of dietary acid ash content.

It has been recommended that a moderate animal protein restriction of 120 gm/day or one gm/kg/day is reasonable for most calcium stone formers. Those patients who ingest large amounts of animal protein should reduce the size of their portions or eliminate meat entirely from some of their meals. A severe protein restriction is not advisable because most patients cannot adhere to such a diet. Similarly, a strict vegetarian diet will reduce the dietary acid ash content, but may also increase oxalate absorption. An increase of citrus fruits and fruit juice in the diet will add an alkaline or antacid load that will help minimize the stone promoting effects of a high acid ash diet. Potassium citrate supplementation will also help to limit the stone promoting effects of excessive dietary acid ash and animal protein.

Dietary Oxalate

Elevated urinary oxalate levels can be a more significant chemical risk factor than a proportionate increase of urinary calcium. Unfortunately, oxalate is so prevalent in the diet that a severe dietary oxalate restriction would be unpalatable. Still, a moderate restriction of those foods with the highest oxalate content is often advisable particularly where there is a history of oxalate stones or elevated urinary oxalate levels. Chocolate, nuts, brewed tea, "sun tea" and green, leafy vegetables have the high bioavailability of oxalate of the items listed. Moderation or restriction of dietary oxalate should always accompany dietary calcium limitations especially in patients with intestinal calcium hyperabsoption. Vitamin C intake beyond 1 gram per day is discouraged because excess Vitamin C may be metabolized to oxalate.

Diet and Kidney Stones

Are all kidney stones the same?

No. Kidney stones are made of different substances and have different causes. The treatment for kidney stones is not the same for everyone.

Is there a diet I can follow to prevent stones? How will I know what diet changes are right for me?

You may need to follow a special diet. First your doctor will need to run tests to find out why you form stones and what diet changes may be right for you. You may be asked to use less salt, calcium, oxalate, or animal protein in your diet. A registered dietitian will be able to plan your diet.

Will following a special diet mean I will not have to take my medicines?

Sometimes, following a special diet may be enough to prevent you from forming more kidney stones. If not, medicines may also need to be taken.

I had a calcium stone. Should I avoid calcium?

Not necessarily. You might put out large amounts of calcium in your urine even if you do not eat high calcium foods. There are special tests that can find out if you need to limit the amount of calcium you eat.

What foods are good sources of calcium?

Dairy products such as milk, cheese, ice cream, and yogurt are high in calcium. Other high calcium foods are sardines or salmon canned with bones, oysters and tofu. Some foods have extra calcium added (for example, some cold cereals and instant oatmeal), and some medicines have large amounts of calcium.

I am worried about developing osteoporosis if I limit the calcium in my diet. How can I protect my bones from becoming weak and brittle as I get older?

You need about 800 to 1000 milligrams of calcium per day. If you eat a diet with less calcium over a long period of time you may have a loss of bone. Most people get about two thirds of their calcium from dairy products. A dietitian can help you to choose the right food to get enough calcium to meet your needs.

My kidney stone contained oxalate. Do I need to avoid all foods high in oxalate?

Sometimes eating foods with a lot of oxalate can make conditions right for you to form a stone. In this case, limiting foods high in oxalate may be helpful. However, totally avoiding foods high in oxalate is not necessary. If your urinary oxalate level is high, then some limitation is reasonable.

What are some of the foods high in oxalate?

Foods with a high content of oxalate include peanuts, peanut butter, tea, rhubarb, beets, spinach and other dark, leafy greens, sweet potato, chocolate, and tofu.

I have had calcium oxalate stones in the past. My doctor tells me to avoid salt. What does salt have to do with calcium oxalate?

A high salt intake can increase the amount of calcium in your urine. Extra calcium in the urine can cause you to form stones. Also, if you are being treated with a thiazide medicine as part of your treatment and you have a high salt intake, the medicine will be less effective.

My doctor told me to drink a lot of fluids. How much is "a lot?" Why is this important?

You should drink at least 12 to 16 cups (3 to 4 quarts or liters) of fluid throughout the day. Most of this should be water. Drinking this amount will allow your kidneys to make at least 2 to 2 $1/2$ quarts of urine—the amount necessary to help prevent new kidney stones. In hot weather you should drink more fluids (above 4 quarts) to make up for fluid lost as sweat. Drinking more fluids should dilute the chemical salts in your urine and prevent their forming a stone. If you live in a hard water area, mention this to the dietitian.

Will it help/hurt me to take a vitamin or mineral supplement?

The B vitamins (which include thiamine, riboflavin, niacin, B-6 and B-12) have not been shown to be harmful to people with kidney stone disease. However, taking vitamin C, vitamin D, fish liver oil, or mineral supplements can increase the chances of stone formation in some people. You should take vitamin and/or mineral supplements ONLY on the advice of your doctor or dietitian.

I've been on preventive therapy for some time now. I just passed another kidney stone. Does this mean the prevention treatment isn't working?

Not necessarily. It's possible that the stone you just passed has been sitting in the kidney since before you even started your prevention treatment. That's why it's important to have an X-ray or other study to verify how many stones are present before starting any stone prevention program. Passing stones that were made before you started the prevention program "don't count." Only the continuing formation of new stones should indicate failure of the prevention program. If this happens, you should be re-tested so appropriate adjustments in your treatment can be started.

Reprinted from The National Kidney Foundation, Inc. Developed by The National Kidney Foundation Council on Renal Nutrition; 1991 04-06NN, Kidney and Urology Facts.

Today the good news is that one does not have to return to the "Stone Age" to prevent kidney stones from occurring. Most physicians simply advise their patients to go back to basics—fresh fruits and vegetables, seeds and whole-grain products, less meat and less fat.

The food charts on the following pages will help you avoid the foods rich in the substances which formed your kidney stone.

Nutrition Charts

Food Sources of Oxalates: Calcium-Oxalate Stones

Fruits	Vegetables	Nuts	Beverages	Other
Berries, all	Baked beans	Almonds	Chocolate	Grits
Currants	Beans, green	Cashews	Cocoa	Tofu, soy
Concord	and wax	Peanuts	Draft beer	products
grapes	Beets	Peanut butter	Tea	Wheat germ
Figs	Beet greens			
Fruit cocktail	Celery			
Plums	Chard, Swiss			
Rhubarb	Chives			
Tangerines	Collards			
	Eggplant			
	Endive			
	Kale			
	Leeks			
	Mustard greens			
	Okra			
	Peppers, green			
	Rutabagas			
	Spinach			
	Squash, summer			
	Sweet potatoes			
	Tomatoes			
	Tomato soup			
	Vegetable soup			

Oxalate Content of Various Foods

FOOD	Mg of Oxalate /100G	MG of Oxalate /serving (serving size in parentheses)
Spinach	645.0	645.0 (100 g)
Fibre One Cereal	142.0	43.0 (30 g)
Bran Flakes	141.0	42.0 (30 g)
Green Beans (steamed)	33.0	33.0 (100 g)
Potato (raw)	27.1	27.1 (100 g)
Butterfinger	53.5	24.0 (45 g)
Peanut Butter	95.8	19.1 (20 g)
Tea (brewed)	7.5	18.8 (250 g)
Celery	61.2	18.4 (30 g)
Chocolate (American)	42.5	13.0 (30 g)
Ravioli	6.5	13.0 (200 g)
White Bread	14.3	8.0 (56 g)
Carrots (raw)	5.7	5.7 (100 g)
Potato Chips	9.4	3.0 (30 g)
White Rice (steamed)	2.1	2.1 (100 g)
Broccoli (steamed)	1.8	1.8 (100 g)
Strawberry jelly	5.3	1.1 (20 g)
Corn Flakes	1.9	0.6 (30 g)
Mustard	12.1	0.6 (5 g)
Apple (raw)	0.5	0.5 (100 g)
Peaches (canned)	0.3	0.3 (100 g)
Grape jelly	1.5	0.3 (20 g)

**Source: Dr. Ross P. Holmes of the Wake Forest University
School of Medicine
Table updated 6/1/98**

Low-Calcium Diet: Calcium Stones
(approximately 400 mg calcium)

	Foods Allowed	Foods Not Allowed
Beverage	Carbonated beverage, coffee, tea	Chocolate-flavored milk, milk drinks
Bread	White and light rye bread or crackers	
Cereals	Refined cereals	Oatmeal, whole-grain cereals
Desserts	Cake, cookies, gelatin desserts, pastries, pudding, sherbets, all made without chocolate; milk or nuts. If egg yolk is used, it must be from one egg allowance.	
Fat	Butter, cream, 2 tbsp daily; French dressing, margarine, salad oil, shortening	Cream (except in amount allowed), mayonnaise
Fruits	Canned, cooked, or fresh fruits or juice except rhubarb	Dried fruit, rhubarb
Meats, eggs	8 oz. daily of any meat, fowl, or fish except clams, oysters, or shrimp; not more than one egg daily including those used in cooking.	Clams, oysters, shrimp, cheese
Potato or substitute	Potato, hominy, macaroni, noodles, refined rice, spaghetti	Whole-grain rice
Soup	Broth, vegetable soup made from vegetables allowed	Bean or pea soup, cream or milk soup
Sweets	Honey, jam, jelly, sugar	
Vegetables	Any canned, cooked, or fresh vegetables or juice except those listed	Dried beans, broccoli, green cabbage, celery, chard, collards, endive, greens, lettuce, lentils, okra, parsley, parsnips, dried peas, rutabagas
Misc.	Herbs, pickles, popcorn, relishes, salt, spices, vinegar	Chocolate, cocoa, milk gravy, nuts, olives, white sauce

Note: Depending on calcium content of local water supply, in instances of high calcium content, distilled water may be indicated.

Low-Calcium Test Diet **
(200 mg calcium)

	Grams	Milligrams Calcium
Breakfast		
Orange Juice, fresh	100	19.00
Bread (toast), white	25	19.57
Butter	15	3.00
Rice Krispies	15	3.70
Cream, 20% butterfat	35	33.95
Sugar	7	0.00
Jam	20	2.00
Distilled water, coffee, or tea*		0.00
TOTAL		**81.22**
Lunch		
Beef steak, cooked	100	10.00
Potato	100	11.00
Tomatoes	100	11.00
Bread	25	19.57
Butter	15	3.00
Honey	20	1.00
Applesauce	20	1.00
Distilled water, coffee or tea		0.00
TOTAL		**56.57**
Dinner		
Lamb chop, cooked	90	10.00
Potato	100	11.00
Frozen green peas	80	10.32
Bread	25	19.57
Butter	15	3.00
Jam	20	2.00
Peach sauce	100	5.00
Distilled water, coffee or tea		0.00
TOTAL		**60.89**

TOTAL MILLIGRAMS CALCIUM   198.68

use distilled water only for cooking and beverages

**Not recommended for long-term use. For testing purposes only.*

Low-Phosphorus Diet: Struvite Stones
(approximately 1 g phosphorus and 40 g protein)

(Struvite stones are composed of a simple compound, magnesium ammonium phosphate (MgNH4PO4). These are often called infection stones because they are associated with urinary tract infections.)

	Foods Allowed	Foods Not Allowed
Milk	Not more than 1 cup daily; whole, skim or buttermilk or 3 tbsp. powered, including the amount used in cooking	Milk and milk drinks except as allowed
Beverages	Fruit juices, tea, coffee, carbonated drinks, Postum	
Bread	White only; enriched commercial, French, hard rolls, soda crackers, rusk	Rye and whole-grain breads, cornbread, biscuits, muffins, waffles
Cereals	Refined cereals, such as Cream of Wheat, Cream of Rice, rice, cornmeal, dry cereals, cornflakes, spaghetti, noodles	All whole-grain cereals
Desserts	Berry or fruit pies, cookies, cakes in average amounts; Jell-O, gelatin, angel food cake, sherbet, meringues made with egg whites, pudding if made with one egg or milk allowance.	Desserts with milk and eggs, unless made with the daily allowance
Eggs	Not more than one egg daily, including those used in cooking; extra egg whites may be used	
Fats	Butter, margarine, oils, shortening	
Fruits	Fresh, frozen, canned, as desired	Dried fruits such as raisins, prunes, dates, figs, apricots

Low-Phosphorus Diet: Struvite Stones
(continued)

	Foods Allowed	Foods Not Allowed
Meat	One large serving or two small servings daily of beef, lamb, veal, pork, rabbit, chicken or turkey	Fish, shellfish (crab, oyster, shrimp, lobster, and so on), dried and cured meats (bacon, ham, chipped beef, and so on), liver, kidney, sweetbreads, brains
Cheese	None	Avoid all cheese and cheese spreads
Vegetables	Potatoes as desired; at least two servings per day of any of the following: asparagus, carrots, beets, green beans, squash, lettuce, rutabagas, tomatoes, celery, peas, onions, cucumber, corn; no more than 1 serving daily of either cabbage, spinach, broccoli, cauliflower, brussel sprouts, or artichokes	Dried vegetables such as peas, mushrooms, lima beans
Misc.	Sugar, jams, jellies, syrups, salt, spices, seasonings; condiments in moderation	

Sample Menu

Breakfast	Lunch	Dinner
Fruit juice	Meat (2 oz.)	Meat (2 oz)
Refined cereal	Potato	Potato
Egg	Vegetable	Vegetable
White toast	Salad	Salad
Butter	Bread, white	Bread, white
1/2 cup milk	Butter	Butter
Coffee or tea	1/2 cup milk	Dessert
	Dessert	Coffee or tea
	Coffee or tea	

Acid Ash Diet: Calcium Stones

The purpose of this diet is to furnish a well-balanced diet in which the total acid ash is greater than the total alkaline ash each day. It lists (1) unrestricted foods, (2) restricted foods, (3) food not allowed, and (4) sample of a day's diet.

Unrestricted Foods
Eat as much as desired of the following foods

Bread any, preferably whole grain, crackers, rolls

Cereals any, preferably whole grain

Desserts angel food or sunshine cake, cookies made without baking powder or soda; cornstarch pudding, cranberry desserts, custards, gelatin desserts, ice cream, sherbet, plum or prune desserts, rice or tapioca pudding

Fats any, as butter, margarine, salad dressings, shortening, lard, salad oils, olive oil

Fruits cranberries, plums, prunes

Meat, eggs, cheese any meat, fish, or fowl, two servings daily; at least one egg daily

Potato substitutes corn, hominy, lentils, macaroni, noodles, rice, spaghetti, vermicelli

Soup broth as desired, other soups from foods allowed

Sweets cranberry or plum jelly; sugar, plain sugar candy

Misc. cream sauce, gravy, peanut butter, peanuts, popcorn, salt, spices, vinegar, walnuts

Restricted Foods
Do not eat any more than the amount allowed each day.

Milk	2 cups daily (may be used in other ways than as beverage) Cream: 1/3 cup or less daily
Fruits	one serving of fruit daily (in addition to prunes, plums, cranberries)
Vegetables including potato	two servings daily; certain vegetables listed under "Foods not allowed" are not allowed at any time.

Foods Not Allowed

	carbonated beverages, such as ginger ale, cola, root beer
	cakes or cookies made with baking powder or soda
Fruits	dried apricots, bananas, dates, figs, raisins, rhubarb
Vegetables	dried beans, beet greens, dandelion greens, carrots, chard, lima beans
Sweets	chocolate or candies other than those under "unrestricted foods;" syrups
Miscellaneous	other than peanuts and walnuts, nuts, olives, pickles

Sample Menu

Breakfast	**Lunch**	**Dinner**
Grapefruit	Creamed chicken	Broth
Wheatena	Steamed rice	Roast beef, gravy
Scrambled eggs	Green beans	Buttered noodles
Toast, butter, plum jam	Stewed prunes	Sliced tomato
Coffee, cream, sugar	Bread, butter	Mayonnaise
	Milk	Bread, butter
		Vanilla ice cream

Low-Purine Foods: Uric Acid Stones

Foods from this list may be used as desired; these foods contain an insignificant amount of purine.

Beverages
Carbonated
Chocolate
Cocoa
Coffee
Fruit juices
Postum
Tea
Butter*
Bread
white and crackers
cornbread
Cereals and cereal products
Corn
Rice
Tapioca
Refined wheat
Macaroni
Noodles
Cheese of all kinds*

Eggs
Fats of all kinds*
(moderation)
Fruits of all kinds
Gelatin, Jell-O®
Milk
buttermilk,
evaporated, malted,
sweet
Nuts of all kinds*,
peanut butter*
Pies*
(except mincemeat)
Sugar and sweets
Vegetables
Artichokes
Beets
Beet greens
Broccoli
Brussels sprouts
Cabbage

Carrots
Celery
Corn
Cucumber
Eggplant
Endive
Kohlrabi
Lettuce
Okra
Parsnips
Potato, white and
sweet
Pumpkin
Rutabagas
Sauerkraut
String beans
Summer squash
Swiss chard
Tomato
Turnips

* high in fat

The foods in the following list contain a moderate amount (up to 75 mg) of purine in 200 g serving. Serve one item four times a week.

Asparagus
Bluefish
Bouillon
Cauliflower
Chicken
Crab
Finnan haddie
Ham

Herring
Kidney beans
Lima beans
Lobster
Mushrooms
Mutton
Navy beans
Oatmeal

Oysters
Peas
Salmon
Shad
Spinach
Tripe
Tuna fish
Whitefish

The following list contains foods that contain a large amount (75-150 mg) of purine in 100 g. serving; one item once a week.

Bacon	Lentils	Quail
Beef	Liver sausage	Rabbit
Calf tongue	Meat soups	Sheep
Carp	Partridge	Shellfish
Chicken Soup	Perch	Squab
Codfish	Pheasant	Trout
Duck	Pigeon	Turkey
Goose	Pike	Veal
Halibut	Pork	Venison

Avoid entirely; foods that contain very large amounts (150-1000 mg) of purine in 100 g serving.

Sweetbreads	825 mg.	Kidneys (beef)	200 mg
Anchovies	363 mg.	Brains	195 mg.
Sardines (in oil)	295 mg.	Meat extracts	(160-400 mg)
Liver (calf, beef)	233 mg.	Gravies	Variable

Typical Meal Pattern

Breakfast	Lunch	Dinner
Fruit	Egg or cheese dish	Egg or cheese dish
Refined cereal and/or egg	Vegetables, as allowed (cooked or salad)	Cream of vegetable soup, if desired
White toast	Potato or substitute	Starch (potato or substitute)
Butter, 1 tsp	White bread	Colored vegetable, as allowed
Sugar	Butter, 1 tsp	White bread
Coffee	Fruit or simple dessert	Butter, 1 tsp if desired
Milk, if desired	Milk	Salad, as allowed
		Fruit or simple dessert
		Milk

Low-Methionine Diet: Cystine Stones

	Foods Allowed	Foods Not Allowed
Soup	Any soup made without meat stock or addition of milk	Rich meat soups, broths, canned soups made with meat broth
Meat or meat substitute	Peanut butter sandwich, spaghetti, or macaroni dish made without addition of meat, cheese, or milk; one serving day day: chicken, lamb, veal, beef, pork, crab, or bacon (3)	Fish and those not listed above
Beverages	Soy milk, tea, coffee	Milk in any form
Vegetables	Asparagus, artichoke, beans, beets, carrots, chicory, cucumber, eggplant, escarole, lettuce, onions, parsnips, potatoes, pumpkin, rhubarb, tomatoes, turnips	Those not listed as allowed
Fruits	Apples, apricots, bananas, berries, cherries, fruit cocktail, grapefruit, grapes, lemon juice, nectarines, oranges, peaches, pears, pineapple, plums, tangerines, watermelon, cantaloupe	Those not listed as allowed
Salads	Raw or cooked vegetable or fruit salad	
Cereals	Macaroni, spaghetti, noodles	
Bread	Whole wheat, rye, white	
Nuts	Peanuts	
Desserts	Fresh or cooked fruit, ices, fruit pies	
Eggs		In any form
Cheese		All varieties
Concentrated sweets	Sugar, jams, jellies, syrup, honey, hard candy	
Concentrated fats	Butter, margarine, cream	
Misc.	Pepper, mustard, vinegar, garlic, oil, herbs, spices	

Meal Pattern

Breakfast	**Lunch**	**Dinner**
1 cup fruit juice	1 serving soup	2 oz. meat
1/2 cup fruit	1 serving sandwich	1 med. starch
1 slice toast	1 cup fruit	1/2 cup vegetable
1 1/2 pats butter	8 oz. soy milk*	1 serving salad
2 tsp jelly	3 tsp sugar	1 tbsp dressing
1 tbsp sugar	1 tbsp cream	1 slice bread
Beverage	Beverage	1 serving dessert
1 tbsp cream		1 tbsp cream
		1 1/2 pats butter
		Beverage

Optional: use for children to include protein intake.
Omit if urine calcium is elevated in adults.

Sample Menu

Breakfast	**Lunch**	**Dinner**
Orange juice	Vegetable soup,	Chicken, roast
Applesauce	vegetarian	Baked potato
Whole-wheat toast	Peanut butter sandwich	Artichoke
Butter	Canned peaches	Sliced tomatoes
Jelly	Soy milk*	French dressing
Sugar	Sugar	Whole-wheat bread
Coffee	Cream	Fruit Ice
Cream	Coffee or tea	Sugar
		Cream
		Butter
		Coffee or tea

Optional: use for children to include protein intake.
Omit if urine calcium is elevated in adults.

Summary of Diet Principles in
Renal Stone Disease

Stone Chemistry	Nutrient Modification	Diet Ash (urinary pH)
Calcium	Low calcium (400 mg)	Acid ash
Phosphate	Low phosphorus (1000 - 1200 mg)	
Oxalate	Low oxalate	
Struvite	Low phosphorus (1000 - 1200 mg) (associated with urinary infections)	Acid ash
Uric acid	Low purine	Alkaline ash
Cystine	Low methionine	Alkaline ash

Adapted from Smith, D.R., Kolb, F.O., and Harper, H.A.: The management of cystinuria and cystine-stone disease. J Urol. 81:61, 1959

Reprinted with permission from Times Mirror/Mosby College Publishing, *Nutrition & Diet Therapy* by Sue Rodwell Williams, Ph.D., M.P.H, R.D., 5th Edition, 1985.

CHAPTER TWENTY

Kidney Stones in Children

Dear Gail:

I recently found out that my six year-old daughter has a kidney stone. I was wondering if you have any info about kidney stones in one that young. My doctor has told me that it is rare.

She had blood drawn yesterday which was a complete nightmare. It took three attempts before they could get the sample. Horrible trauma for her. I had told the nurse that she could not "stick" her again—so it was a good thing she finally got it!

She had a renal sonogram today. I won't have the results of either the blood work or the sonogram back until next week.

She did have a pretty painful bout on Sunday evening. She screamed for about 55 minutes straight...clutching her crotch the entire time. She is terrified of going to the bathroom. I'm not sure how much of the screaming was related to the pain and how much was related to fatigue. We were on the road in the middle of nowhere...or she would have been at an ER immediately. By the time we got close to a hospital, she had fallen asleep so we took her on home rather than waking her for more poking and prodding in the middle of the night. Since then, she has been relatively happy. She is insistent on wearing pull-ups rather than panties because she is convinced that she can potty in the pull-ups and it won't hurt her as bad as if she tries to use the toilet.

Among my most heart-rending letters—and phone calls—are those from anguished parents whose young children have kidney stones. These special little patients are always described as "Real Troopers." They endure procedures that would leave most adults in a cold sweat. Hugging favorite teddy bears or other stuffed animals, braving medical offices dressed in pajamas meant for sleep-overs at friends' homes, these littlest stone sufferers deserve Purple Hearts. I have found that parents are often reluctant to put their child through just one more test or to make "one more phone call and try this new urologist." These young patients have been pushed to the extreme, and their parents as well.

Statistically, pediatric stone disease, defined as kidney stones occurring before 16 years of age, constitutes only about seven percent of the total urinary stone population. If it happens to your child, however, statistics don't matter. You need immediate information.

In infants, pain from stones may mimic colic. But fortunately stones are extremely uncommon in infants under age two, or in Black children.

Metabolic problems in children tend to be more severe than in adults and are more likely to require aggressive therapy. Unlike adults, there is no gender difference: kidney stones are equally distributed between girls and boys. Stone recurrence rates in children range from 16 to 44 percent.

Until about 1980, most experts believed that the underlying cause of most stones in children was urinary blockage, congenital or inherited problems, anomalies in basic anatomy or urinary infections. Since then, many studies have demonstrated that at least two-thirds of pediatric stone patients have a specific, identifiable, underlying chemical or metabolic disorder. Most experts now recommend long-term observation and metabolic testing for all children who form even one kidney stone.

The highest new stone formation rates are due to metabolic causes in people living in the "Stone Belt" parts of the country, roughly the entire Southern half of the United States. There is a relatively high rate of family stone disease with 20 to 37 percent of pediatric stone formers having a family history for stones.

Children with urinary stones have many of the same medical problems as adults, including hyperparathyroidism, cystinuria, renal tubular acidosis, low urinary citrate, high urinary oxalate, low urinary volume, high uric acid, and high urinary calcium.

High urinary calcium can cause either visible or just microscopic blood in the urine of children even without obvious stones. This is thought to be due to microscopic crystals forming inside the kidney that damage the cells lining the urinary system.

The presence of high urinary calcium in the urine eventually leads to calcium stone disease in 20 percent of children within five years. This is more likely due to renal calcium leak rather than increased intestinal calcium absorption, which is exactly the opposite of adults. High urinary calcium has also been identified as a cause of painful, urgent, and/or frequent urination. Interestingly, a very large percentage of children with both blood traces in their urine and a family history of kidney stones have high urinary calcium. Of this group, roughly equal portions had increased intestinal calcium absorption and renal calcium leak.

Calcium excretion in babies is strongly influenced by the type of milk the baby drinks. Breast milk is associated with a higher urinary calcium excretion, perhaps because of the low phosphorus content of human milk. Soy-based formulas produce the lowest urinary calcium excretion. Preliminary evidence suggests that urinary calcium also may be somewhat elevated during adolescence.

Prolonged use of Lasix (furosemide), a common medication used to increase urine production, has been associated with kidney stones in premature infants. In such patients, Lasix can increase calcium excretion 10 to 20 times and has a prolonged half-life (which means that the medicine lasts much longer in the body than normal). Thiazide therapy significantly lowers urinary calcium levels and occasionally dissolves stones formed while under furosemide treatment. Lasix induced stone disease is five times more prevalent in the Caucasian population. There doesn't appear to be any permanent damage beyond 8 months of age in infants who had formed stones while on Lasix therapy.

High urinary uric acid in children is associated with a variety of medical conditions. For example, high cell turnover rates due to chemotherapy or leukemia can cause uric acid stones in up to 50 percent of affected children. In addition, disorders of protein digestion can lead to abnormally high levels of uric acid. And certain drugs such as X-ray contrast media, probenecid, colchicine and aspirin-related medications can increase urinary uric acid levels.

Children with cystic fibrosis receiving large oral doses of pancreatic enzymes may develop increased uric acid and urinary calcium levels. They also have low urinary citrate and magnesium levels.

However, while there is substantial evidence that high urinary uric acid increases calcium oxalate stone formation in adults, it doesn't appear to be a significant risk factor for calcium stones in children. Only 4 percent of pediatric urinary stones are composed of uric acid.

The most common cause of low urinary citrate levels in children is renal tubular acidosis. In this condition, there is a failure of the kidney to excrete extra acid. This is always accompanied by very low levels of urinary citrate. Abnormally high urinary calcium may also be present. Supplemental oral citrate is the preferred therapy.

Stone Therapy for Children

At least fifty percent of children with stones will pass the stones without intervention or surgery. Cases requiring surgery are similar to those for adults:

- Uncontrollable pain.

- Persistent blockage of the kidney with risk for permanent damage.

- Clear evidence of stone growth.

- Persistent urinary infection.

While virtually all surgical procedures used for adults are available for children, the treatment of choice is lithotripsy (ESWL). This can be used quite successfully.

Stone Prevention in Children

Preventive therapy in children is often difficult. The initial treatment for high urinary calcium is to drink more fluids and eat less salt. If this fails, oral thiazide therapy is usually effective. Potassium citrate and orthophosphates have also been used with success.

Dietary calcium restrictions are usually not considered appropriate in growing children due to concerns about normal growth patterns, bone density growth, and possible increase in oxalate absorption from the intestinal tract. Urinary alkalinization with potassium citrate is usually sufficient to prevent uric acid stones. Extremely high uric acid in either the urine or blood requires allopurinol, a prescription medication.

High urinary oxalate is rare in children. When present, it can be treated with a low oxalate diet, Vitamin B-6 and calcium citrate. The supplemental calcium binds strongly to oxalate in the intestinal tract, limiting oxalate absorption. Calcium citrate is the preferred calcium supplement for this purpose because it's the least likely calcium product to promote calcium stone formation.

CHAPTER TWENTY-ONE

A Note to Kids Whose Parents Have Stones
—From a Kid Who Knows—

By Jennifer Golomb

Hi! My name is Jennifer Golomb and I am Gail's daughter. I thought it was important to have a "word" with kids who have a Mom or Dad who has kidney stones because it affects the whole family and it is scary to see your parent in a lot of pain. I am now 19 years-old.

I was 10 years old when my mom went to the hospital emergency room with a kidney stone. Until that time I never even knew what stones were, let alone know that we had kidneys. The closest thing I knew about kidneys was there was something named kidney beans and my brother loved to eat them, but to me they didn't smell too good.

When my mother had her first stone, I thought I was the one having a mid-life crisis, just like the adult game with that name. I thought I was the only kid in the universe with problems. From that time on, I was afraid that I would wake up one morning and my mom would be in the hospital again instead of at home with me. It frightened me so much that I can still vividly remember those days as if they were yesterday.

I recall a year after her first episode, Mom was in the hospital and her friend was at home taking care of me. I expected my mom. There were times when I thought my mom would die. What did I know? I was just a kid. When Mom was in that much pain, there was no one to explain things to me.

I was very scared and I felt very much alone.

My mom helped me put a smile on my face when two days after she had been to the emergency room she took me out to get my favorite ice cream in a waffle cone. She explained to me what stones were, how they leave the body and why there was so much pain, and what she could do to prevent new stones from forming. She said she thought she might even write a book about kidney stones! Even though I spent most of my time fishing out the biggest chocolate chip pieces I could find in the ice cream, her talk made me feel a lot better.

"Truth" is the hardest word in the English language, but it is the most important word to follow! Parents should always tell their children the truth when it comes to kidney stones.

Jennifer Golomb
Author's daughter

I love my mom and I usually know when something is wrong—if she is in pain or not feeling too well. I like to be told what I can do to help. When I was little, I wanted to know what would happen to my brother and myself if Mom had to go to the hospital. The very, very most important thing for a parent to say is that "I will not die" from a kidney stone because that is the very first thing us kids think. Also, tell your kid you love them (whether they're big or small!).

Parents should let their children know that millions of children go through this experience each year with a parent. Kidney stones are a family experience and everyone needs to help. Since stones can be prevented, there is absolutely no reason to put a child through such fear and terror watching a parent terrorized by horrific pain.

My mom taught me some important things since her kidney stones. We are now a family that drinks a lot of water together. Mom likes to laugh that "a family that drinks water together, stays together." She has taught me and my brother to do a lot of water drinking. And if we see that one of us is not drinking water, the other person brings it to their attention. This is how we show that we love each other.

Here is a list of some things a kid can do to help their parent:

1. You can put on a funny play for your parent to make them laugh.

2. Make a pretty get-well card.

3. You can clean up the house for your Mom or Dad. They don't feel well anyway and this is extra special to do.

4. Ask them if there is anything you can do, and if they want to sleep—let your Mom or Dad sleep.

5. When they feel better, make them a peanut butter and jelly sandwich (as long as that doesn't make another kidney stone!) and serve it with a tall glass of milk!

6. Bring them a glass of water to drink before they ask for one! In fact, bring them two glasses of water to drink!

7. Some kids might think this is gross...but you ought to see what a kidney stone looks like. I didn't think our body could make that kind of stone. I took it to my science class. The teacher showed the rest of the students. He made us drink more water. But most of the students wanted to anyway after they saw that stone!

8. Bring your parent a stone or a special rock from outside and make a joke out of it. You know—kidney "stone."

9. Go food shopping with your parent and take along the food chapter from my mom's book. Make sure your parent doesn't buy any foods which could make them form a new kidney stone. Find a new food to eat instead of the "bad" food.

10. It's important to take care of yourself, too, even if you are a kid because with some kidney stones, if your mom or dad has one, then someday you can get one! I try to drink lots of water. Teach this to your little brothers and sisters.

11. Learn where your kidneys are located. Have your doctor or pediatrician point them out to you.

12. If you go out for a sport, be sure to increase how much water you drink. Make sure your team drinks a lot of water, too.

13. Most importantly, tell your parent how much you love them! That can be the best medicine in the world.

14. Make sure your dog or cat drinks a lot of water. Some of them get kidney and bladder stones, too.

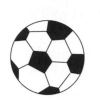

**Good luck,
Jennifer**

CHAPTER TWENTY-TWO

Important Medical References to Read and Show Your Doctor

The following is a listing of some of the more important and readable medical references on kidney stone disease and prevention. You can obtain them from your nearest hospital medical library. While not designed for the general public, if you have gotten this far in this book you now probably know more than most physicians about kidney stone disease and are ready for this new challenge. Use the Glossary to help you with some of the medical terminology.

The other use of this material is to help you convince your doctor and even your insurance company if necessary of the medical prudence and cost effectiveness of stone prevention programs.

BIBLIOGRAPHY

Begun, F., Foley, D., Peterson, A. and White, B.: Patient Evaluation: Laboratory and Imaging Studies, Urologic Clinics of North America, Vol. 24, No. 1, pp. 97 - 116, February 1997

Curhan, G., Willett, W., Rimm, E. and Stampfer, M.: A Prospective Study of Dietary Calcium and Other Nutrients and the Risk of Symptomatic Kidney Stones, New England Journal of Medicine, Vol. 328, No. 12, pp. 833 - 838, 1993

Leslie, S.: Outpatient Metabolic Evaluation of Patients With Recurrent Kidney Stones, OHIO Medicine: Journal of the Ohio State Medical Association, Vol. 185, No. 4, pp. 292 - 294, 1989

NIH Consensus Conference: Prevention and Treatment of Kidney Stones, Journal of the American Medical Association, Vol. 260, pp. 978 - 981, 1988

Pak, C.: Role of Medical Prevention, Journal of Urology, Vol. 141, pp. 798 - 800, 1989

Pak, C.: The Many Facets of Kidney Stone Disease, Contemporary Urology, pp. 56 - 62, January/February 1990

Parivar, F., Low, R., and Stoller, M.: The Influence of Diet on Urinary Stone Disease, Journal of Urology, Vol. 155, pp. 432 - 440, 1996

Parks, J. and Coe, F.: The Financial Effects of Kidney Stone Prevention, Kidney International, Vol. 50, pp. 1706 - 1712, 1996

Preminger, G., Peterson, R., Peters, P. and Pak, C.: The Current Role of Medical Treatment of Nephrolithiasis: The Impact of Improved Techniques of Stone Removal, Journal of Urology, Vol. 134, pp. 6 - 10, 1985

Resnick, M. and Pak, C.: Editorial: Are Metabolic Studies of Urolithiasis Necessary?, Journal of Urology, Vol. 137, pp. 960 - 961, 1987

Ruml, L., Pearle, M. and Pak, C: Medical Therapy of Calcium Oxalate Urolithiasis, Urologic Clinics of North America, Vol. 24, No. 1 pp. 117 - 133, February 1997

Segura, J., Preminger, G., Assimos, D., et al: Nephrolithiasis Clinical Guidelines Panels: Report on the Management of Staghorn Calculi, Journal of Urology, Vol. 151, pp. 1648 - 1651, 1994

CHAPTER TWENTY-THREE

Questions and Answers

Why Do Kidney Stones Hurt So Much?

A kidney stone pain attack, also called **"colic"**, is described as the most painful experience it's possible to live through. It's more painful than gunshot wounds, major surgery, broken bones, burns and even childbirth. The pain is unrelated to the size of the stone and is not caused by the stone "moving" or scratching as many people believe. In fact, the pain is caused by the dilating or stretching and cramping of the urinary system caused by the blockage the stone produces when it gets stuck in the ureter. (The ureter is the muscular tube that drains urine from the kidneys into the urinary bladder.)

When the urine that the kidney produces cannot pass the blockage, the ureter and urinary system stretch. The ureter is composed of muscle and will contract or cramp when stretched. This stretching, dilating and cramping is what causes the intense pain. (The same process causes the pain from intestinal gas that we all get from time to time.) This also explains why the stones usually don't cause pain when they are just sitting inside the kidney. Since they don't produce any blockage, stretching or dilating of the urinary system, they don't usually produce any pain until they pass out of the kidney and get stuck.

The degree of pain is unrelated to the size of the stone which is why it is possible to have excruciating pain from a stone smaller than a grain of rice. Typically, the pain will start in the upper back on the side of the affected kidney. The pain will then travel or radiate down and around the flank or side and head towards the groin. Most people can correctly identify the exact site of their stone just by pointing to where the pain is worst.

Fortunately, many small stones will pass without the patient even knowing it. The pain from a stone attack, even when very severe, will usually pass in about 24 hours. This is because the urinary system will reach a point where some urine sneaks around the obstructing stone and the stretching and cramping will stop.

Just because the pain may go away does not necessarily mean that the stone is gone. Usually an X-ray will be needed to determine if in fact the stone is still present or not. Stones can fragment in the system so even if you pass one "stone" another fragment may remain inside.

In the past, patients with colic were routinely admitted to the hospital so they could receive strong pain medicine usually by injection. Now we only bring patients into the hospital when we cannot manage their pain adequately with oral medications alone or if there is a potential complication such as an infection, a solitary kidney or a pregnancy. Even then, patients often stay only 24 hours or less in the hospital on "observation" status. Fortunately, most patients do not have to stay in the hospital very long and many can be safely sent home from the Emergency Room once a diagnosis is made and initial treatment begun.

Some stones will get stuck in such a way that they will cause an intermittent problem. This is sometimes called a "ball-valve" since the pain can and usually does return quickly between attacks. Since no equalization occurs, this type of intermittent pain attack can continue much longer than 24 hours.

There are three areas in the urinary system where stones are most likely to get stuck and cause a blockage. The first is just where the central collection sack of the kidney joins with the top of the **ureter**. (The ureter is the muscular tube that drains urine from the kidney to the urinary bladder.) This area is called the Ureteropelvic Junction or "UPJ". This structure is normally a wide open funnel shaped cone, but some people are born with an anatomical narrowing at this point. Stones that get stuck here will probably get stuck somewhere else downstream, so we often will try to do some treatment of the stone relatively quickly. Stones can be blasted with "ESWL" easily here, although the best location for ESWL is in the kidney itself. (Actually, it's possible to use ESWL on any part of the urinary system, but most experts agree that the kidney is the ideal stone location.)

The next area of increased risk is about two thirds of the way down the ureter towards the bladder. This is where the ureter bends to pass over the large blood vessels taking blood to the legs. The narrowest part of the ureter is where it attaches to the bladder itself. This is called the Ureterovesical Junction or "UVJ". The ureter passes through the muscular wall of the bladder at a steep angle. This anatomy works as a valve to keep urine from backing up into the ureter every time the bladder contracts during voiding. Even a relatively small stone here can easily become stuck. Irritation of the bladder wall will cause many people to have cramps or spasms of the bladder and urinary frequency if a stone is stuck here.

If a stone is not causing any blockage and there is no infection, then there will not be any pain from that stone. There must be blockage or infection for a stone to cause pain. Sometimes, just after a stone has passed, there will be some residual inflammation and partial blockage. In these cases there can be some temporary pain or discomfort. But in general, there must be either obstruction to the urinary system or infection for a stone to cause pain.

What Is A Stent And Will I Need One?

A stent is a slender, plastic tube placed within the urinary system. One end sits in the central part of the kidney where the urine collects and the other end is in the bladder. It is completely internal. Its function is to guarantee drainage of the kidney, provide support to the ureter, improve visualization of any hard to see stones, bypass any obstructive stone or scar tissue and relieve pain.

Your urologist will decide whether you need one after reviewing your X-rays and evaluating your individual situation. The decision on your need for a stent can be very technical because there are many factors to consider. We recommend that you let your urologist make this decision, but be sure to ask him the specific reasons.

Usually stents are intended for short term use but occasionally they need to remain longer. The maximum time a stent can be in the body should probably be no more than 6 months because of the possibility of forming stones and clogging the stent. Dr. Leslie has seen stents that have become completely encased in stone material because they were not removed until well after the recommended time period.

Will My Stone Pass Without Surgery?

If the stone is 4 mm or less, then there is a 90 percent chance of spontaneous passage. Stones 5 mm (about 1/4 inch) to 7 mm in size have a 50 percent chance of passing, while stones larger than 7 mm only rarely pass by themselves. Whenever possible, we like to give the stone every chance to pass by itself before resorting to surgery.

What Are My Chances of Having Another Stone Attack?

If there are no additional stones in your kidneys now and this was your first stone attack, then your chances of forming another stone is about 10% a year although this will vary according to the specific chemical problems that are involved with each individual patient. Younger patients and those with a close family member or blood relative with stones are at greater risk. The peak ages for kidney stone production are between twenty and forty years of age. On the average, the risk of having another stone problem if you've just had your first stone attack is about 70-80%. If you live in the "Stone Belt", then your chances will be higher. As a white male, your chance of having at least one stone by age 70 is one out of eight.

Can't You Dissolve The Stone With Medicine?

Unfortunately, most stones are made of a variety of calcium mineral combinations that can't be dissolved with any known medicine. About 10% of all stones are made up of uric acid. Only these pure uric acid stones can sometimes be dissolved with proper medication. The majority of stones are made of calcium which cannot be dissolved. We do have many methods for getting rid of kidney stones relatively painlessly, such as ESWL which stands for Extracorporeal Shock Wave Lithotripsy.

If I Get A Stone Attack, What Should I Do?

It may not be easy to tell if you're having a kidney stone attack or some other potentially serious medical problem. The best policy is to go directly to a hospital emergency room. (Urgent care centers and physician's offices may not have the diagnostic testing available to make a definitive diagnosis and you might end up being transferred after much delay to a hospital anyway.) Only about 50% of the cases of severe flank and abdominal pain that start out as possible kidney stone attacks actually turn out to be true stone events! The rest can be other medical problems such as appendicitis, bowel disease, intestinal obstruction, ulcers, abscesses and a variety of other medical diseases and conditions. (See section on Diagnosis)

There are several symptoms that clearly indicate the need to go to the hospital.

■ Severe pain not controlled by oral pain medication.

■ High fever.

■ Persistent vomiting.

■ Unable to take oral fluids.

■ Severe or persistent diarrhea.

■ History of a solitary kidney, kidney failure or pregnancy.

You cannot make the diagnosis of kidney stones yourself. Even if you're sure the pain is identical to your last stone attack, you could be wrong and have to suffer the consequences if it just happens to be your appendix. **Always have the problem checked by a physician!**

What About Using The "Stone Machine" To Break It Up?

The "Stone Machine" or ESWL, fragments stones by using shock waves. The original machine produced shock waves with a special spark plug located at the bottom of a tank of water. These shock waves are then focused at a predetermined spot in the tank. The patient is anesthetized and placed on a special frame which is lowered into the tank. The patient and frame are then gently maneuvered inside the tank until the stone is positioned precisely at the focal point of the shock waves. X-rays are used to pinpoint the location of the stone and to make certain it remains exactly at the correct spot. The shock waves literally vibrate the stone so intensely it eventually shatters and fragments without injury to the surrounding tissues. In order to use the machine, the stone needs to be large enough to be seen clearly under the X-rays used for positioning. The stone also has to be in a location such as the kidney where the shock waves can reach it easily without striking bone.

Many newer machines have eliminated the water tank and do not require full anesthesia. Most of these newer machines are not as powerful as the original so there is a greater chance that a second treatment will be needed before all the stone material is completely fragmented.

It may take three months or longer to pass all the stone fragments after a successful treatment and there is a weight limitation on most available machines of 300 pounds. Patients who weigh more may not be able to use this technology.

Which Jobs Or Professions Are The Most Dangerous When Associated With Kidney Stones?

It's well established that professional airline pilots can't fly if they have a known kidney stone until it either passes or is removed. Military personnel who are stationed in warm climates around the world, such as Navy seamen on an aircraft carrier, would also have above average risk because they are generally in the peak age group for stone production and are far away from the nearest ESWL stone blasting machine.

People who work in submarines that are out of touch will be at high risk for the same reason. To me, the greatest risk would be to astronauts. Not only does space flight cause chemical changes that lead to stones, such as decreased stone blockers like citrate and increased stone promoters like calcium and uric acid, but there is absolutely no way they can get immediate medical help. This has happened on several NASA shuttle missions and to Russian cosmonauts. The most famous case occurred on Apollo 13 where one of the astronauts on the way to the moon got a stone attack (that was also the mission where the service module exploded and they had to circle the moon to turn around and come back to earth).

What Kind of Diet Should I Eat To Avoid More Stones?

This is probably the question we get asked most often. There is no easy answer to what type of diet you should follow. It depends on the type of stones you are making and the chemical abnormalities and risk factors your body produces. The only way to tell for sure is to analyze any stones or stone fragments that have been collected **and** to perform a comprehensive blood and urine chemical testing series designed to show the specific problems in your particular case. Then, specific recommendations can be made.

However, if you really need an answer, we can make a few general recommendations. First, drink more water and fluids. There was probably not enough urinary volume to dissolve all the chemicals the kidneys were trying to get rid of at some point. Secondly, as far as the rest of the diet, the best advice is to avoid excess in all the types of food you eat. Excessive salt, fat and meat protein should probably be avoided. But with fifty separate potential stone composition chemicals and over sixty five different medical problems, conditions, deficiencies, excesses or disorders that can contribute to stone disease, it's easy to see that no single piece of advice is likely to help every situation. Therefore, we urge every patient interested in preventing stones to get properly tested and treated by a physician interested and knowledgeable in kidney stone disease prevention.

Why Limit Salt (Sodium) And Meat Protein?

Excess dietary salt (sodium) will tend to promote kidney stone formation primarily by increasing urinary calcium excretion. Sodium changes the way that calcium is handled by the kidneys. The higher the sodium load, the greater the amount of calcium that will appear in the urine. It may also decrease urinary citrate, an important kidney stone inhibitor.

Excessive meat protein in the diet will tend to increase urinary calcium, oxalate and uric acid levels as well as make the urine more acid. All of these changes will increase the risk of kidney stones. When meat protein is fully digested, it tends to leave an acid residue which is excreted by the kidneys. Uric acid is a waste product made from the chemical digestion of purines, a component of the genetic code material inside all living cells. Those proteins that have high levels of purine will create higher levels of uric acid. These high purine proteins are red meat, poultry and fish. Vegetable protein has much lower levels of purine than animal protein. Uric acid can form stones by itself and promote the creation of calcium stones by forming tiny crystals or stones which quickly become covered with calcium compounds in susceptible people. Some stone patients will stop making stones if they can simply control their excessive dietary meat protein intake.

What About Just Limiting My Intake of Calcium and Dairy Products?

Many kidney stone patients severely restrict their calcium intake without realizing that such a reduction in dietary calcium can actually increase their risk of calcium stone disease. Dietary calcium has an important role to play in binding other minerals within the intestinal tract. A significant reduction in calcium intake can cause an increase in absorption of some of these other minerals which are normally bound or attached to the calcium. When not enough calcium is available for these minerals to bind to, they are left free to be absorbed by the body and eventually excreted in the urine where they can help form new stones. The net result is an increase in the risk of forming more calcium stones if calcium intake is restricted too severely!

Dairy products not only contain a relatively large amount of calcium, but they are also rich in phosphate and magnesium, two important kidney stone formation blockers. Eliminating dairy products would therefore cause a decrease in these two important stone prevention chemicals.

Finally, when you eliminate calcium from the diet, the intestinal tract attempts to compensate by increasing the rate or percentage of calcium absorption. (Normally, we only absorb 30-45% of the calcium we eat.) If you should "cheat" and actually eat a high calcium meal when the intestinal tract is in this higher absorption, sensitized condition, the amount of calcium actually entering the body would be much higher than normal. A sudden calcium load may begin the formation of a new kidney stone.

How Can I Avoid Getting More Kidney Stones?

While we have excellent methods of fragmenting stones with shock wave machines, lasers and internal lithotriptors, it's much more efficient and cost effective to eliminate the true, underlying causes of kidney stone formation whenever possible.

The first essential step in the prevention of kidney stones is to guarantee that there will always be sufficient water intake to produce enough urine to easily dissolve all the minerals and chemicals the kidneys normally produce and excrete. In other words, if you could drink enough water and liquids to always keep the chemical and mineral content of the urine from becoming too concentrated, you would never form any kidney stones. Without sufficient fluid intake, no prevention program has any chance of success.

In general, we recommend increasing fluid intake throughout the day and dietary moderation of most food groups. Patients should also avoid excessive dietary intake of dairy products (calcium), meat and salt.

The only way to identify the specific chemical or mineral imbalances that contribute to kidney stone formation in any individual patient is to perform a comprehensive series of blood and urine chemistry tests. This preventive testing series, called **Metabolic Analysis or Metabolic Testing**, is absolutely essential in order to identify the specific risk factors in a particular patient. Knowing the chemical composition of any previous kidney stones or stone fragments is extremely helpful, but without a Metabolic Testing Program it is impossible to identify the particular cause of an individual's production of stones.

Therapy usually consists of various but specific dietary adjustments or nutritional supplements. Sometimes medication is required when dietary treatment alone has failed to correct the chemical imbalance. The patient must be motivated to follow treatment suggestions for an indefinite period for any prevention program to be ultimately successful.

Conservative treatment measures such as dietary moderation and increasing fluid intake can reduce recurrences by about 60 percent. Metabolic Testing consisting of comprehensive blood and urine chemistry analysis, together with a specific treatment plan can reduce the risk of new stone formation by up to 98 percent!

What Exactly Is Involved In Metabolic Testing For Stone Prevention?

Comprehensive blood and urine chemical testing is needed to identify the specific risk factors in kidney stone formation for any individual patient. 24 hour urine collections are required along with a blood test. These samples are then tested extensively to uncover any predisposing chemical problem that could lead to kidney stone formation. Any stone material that has been passed must be recovered to be chemically analyzed. This will help in developing a treatment plan to prevent more kidney stones from forming. Insurance usually covers the cost of the metabolic testing. Excellent stone prevention testing programs are available nationally at reasonable cost, but they will require a physician's order to obtain (see pages 109 - 111).

What Are The Most Common Problems Found In Metabolic Testing?

The five most common problems are high uric acid, low urinary citrate, low urinary volume, high urinary calcium and high urinary oxalate. Each is found in roughly 20-35 percent of patients tested. It's not possible to predict which types of problems will be encountered just by the X-ray appearance of the stone or even with the stone chemical composition. That's why the blood and urine chemistry testing is essential to identify the high risk factors responsible for stone production in each individual patient. While these are the most common problems, there are many other possible chemical risk factors that should be included when testing is performed.

Who Should Receive Metabolic Testing For Stones?

We strongly recommend metabolic testing for patients with multiple stone attacks, especially if at a young age. There is general agreement that all children with kidney stones should be tested. Beyond that, it's a question of motivation and risk. Someone strongly motivated to follow a treatment plan for an indefinite period if it will reduce their risk of new stones probably should be tested even if they only had a single stone. Others with less motivation to follow preventive treatment would probably not benefit much from the evaluation even if they have very active disease. A certain minimal evaluation to identify obvious medical disorders probably should be done on every stone patient.

How Can I Stay Motivated To Follow A Prevention Plan?

The real motivation has to come from you. How badly do you want to avoid more stones? How much pain did that last stone give you? For most people, the memory of an intense pain like a stone attack fades quickly. One way to remember how bad the stone episode was is to write yourself a note or postcard. Whenever you feel like quitting the program, just look at the note. You need to remind yourself just how bad the pain and discomfort was.

What is a Ammonium Urate Stone?

Ammonium urate is a relatively rare type of kidney stone. People who make this type of stone are almost always abusing laxatives. The condition is characterized by low urinary volume, high urinary acidity, low serum potassium, low urinary citrate and highurinary ammonia. All of these chemical problems are directly related to excess laxative use which causes the loss of fluid, bicarbonate and potassium through the intestinal tract.

This condition is most common in women who usually are thin and anorexic. The ammonium urate stones may be associated with uric acid and calcium oxalate stones. This condition is a psychological problem caused by the laxative abuse. Once the abnormal laxative use is resolved, stone production stops.

What are Nanobacteria?

Nanobacteria are the smallest known bacteria. These highly resistant organisms normally produce calcium phosphate crystals on their surface. These microcrystals could be the first step in kidney stone production. In one study, 30 kidney stones were meticulously examined for nanobacteria. All of the stone studies were positive for the organisms. Someday we may use special antibiotics to help prevent stones caused by these newly discovered nanobacteria.

CHAPTER TWENTY-FOUR

List of Medications

ACE Inhibitor

A type of high blood pressure medicine which may decrease urinary citrate. ACE stands for Angiotension Converting Enzyme. This type of medication blocks the activity of an enzyme which would otherwise create chemicals in the body that would increase the blood pressure.

Allopurinol

Blocks the formation of uric acid in humans. This forces the body to make an alternate chemical called xanthine which is easier to dissolve than uric acid. This medication is often used in pure uric acid stones, gout or whenever the uric acid levels in the blood or urine need to be reduced.

Aluminum Hydroxide

This is occasionally used in patients with Struvite or infection stones to help bind intestinal phosphate and limit its absorption. It's also used as a substitute oxalate binding agent where calcium is not appropriate.

Aluminum Hydroxide (continued)

Tends to cause constipation. Cannot be used in patients with kidney failure because of possibly dangerous accumulations in the body.

Amiloride

A type of potassium sparing "water pill" or diuretic.

Beelith

A magnesium supplement.

Bucillamine

Experimental drug that increases dissolvability of cystine. Expected to be more effective with fewer side effects than penicillamine.

Calcitriol

Another name for activated Vitamin D or Vitamin D3.

Calcitonin

Hormone that increases calcium deposition in bone and is generally the exact opposite of parathyroid hormone.

Calcium Citrate

The preferred type of calcium supplement for kidney stone formers. The extra citrate helps avoid any increase in calcium stone formation.

Captopril

A blood pressure medicine which is thought to be able to bind with cystine and make it more dissolvable. While safe and well tolerated, its effectiveness in cystine stone disease is unclear.

Cellulose

A strong binder of calcium in the digestive tract.

Cholestyramine

A strong binding agent for oxalate in the intestinal tract. Takes the place of calcium in enteric hyperoxaluria. Effective, but tends to have side effects.

Codeine
An oral pain medication of medium strength. An opioid

Demerol
A strong Opioid type of pain medication.

Diamox (Acetazolamide)
Normally used for glaucoma, this medication will block excretion of acid from the kidneys and alkalinize the urine. Can be of use in severe cystinuria, but generally should be avoided in most stone patients if possible.

Dilantin
A medicine commonly used for seizures. Can interfere with Vitamin D activity.

Diuretic
A type of medication that causes the kidneys to make more urine. Can be used to increase urinary volume but only as a last resort. Some diuretics, like thiazide, can be used to help decrease stone disease while others cannot. Originally intended as therapy for blood pressure and heart failure.

Diuril
A common thiazide medication.

Dyazide
A high blood pressure medication composed of a thiazide and triamterene. Should not be used in stone patients because triamterene can sometimes form kidney stones by itself!

Elmiron (Pentosan Polysulfate)
Originally designed as a therapy for interstitial cystitis, an unusual inflammatory condition of the urinary bladder. This medication restores the normal mucus coating of the bladder lining. There is evidence

Elmiron (continued)

that Elmiron can be a strong inhibitor of calcium oxalate stone formation, but only limited human studies are available at this time. Still, it could be of some use in the most severe and intractable cases of high urinary oxalate.

Estrogen

A female hormone. Will increase calcium in bone.

Fosamax

A new class of medication that is designed for osteoporosis. Works almost as good as estrogen in replacing calcium in bone.

Hydrochlorothiazide

The standard thiazide medication. Usually not the preferred agent in stone disease because it must be taken twice a day while other thiazides like Naqua and Lozol only need to be taken once daily.

Lithostat (Acetohydroxamic Acid or AHA)

Blocks the chemical released by bacteria that allows struvite stones to form. Has moderate side effects so must be used carefully.

Lozol (Indapamide)

A long acting water pill (diuretic) that has an almost identical function to thiazide but is not technically one of them. Will also take calcium out of the urine and return it to the bloodstream. Only needs to be taken once a day.

Magnesium Oxide (Beelith) and Magnesium Hydroxide

Common magnesium supplements.

Moduretic	Combination of thiazide and amiloride. The amiloride returns potassium to the blood that would otherwise be lost. Needs to be taken twice a day. A good substitute for Dyazide.
Morphine	A strong opioid type of pain medication; usually requires an injection.
Naqua (trichlormethiazide)	A long acting thiazide. Only needs to be taken once a day.
Nubain	A potent pain medicine used for severe pain. Requires injection, not an opioid. Roughly equal to Morphine.
Opioid	A group of medicines chemically related to extracts from opium. Morphine and Codeine are examples.
Orthophosphate	An oral form of phosphate supplement.
Oxythiozolidine (OZT)	An experimental medication that decreases liver production of oxalate by about one third.
Percocet and Percodan	Oral tablets of a moderately strong Opioid medication.
Penicillamine	A binding agent for cystinuria. Side effects are severe and common. Only about 50 percent of patients with cystinuria can tolerate this medication even though it is very effective.
Persantine	Can somewhat reduce the excessive loss of phosphate in Renal Phosphate Leak.

Polycitra K A liquid form of potassium citrate. Also available as crystals in a packet than can be mixed with water or juice.

Potassium Magnesium Citrate Experimental form of citrate supplement. Not only provides high citrate boost to the urine, but also benefits stone prevention by adding the magnesium supplement. Will probably be the replacement for Urocit-K when it becomes available.

Prednisone The most common oral steroid. A very effective anti-inflammatory, but has several side effects.

Pyridoxine Another name for Vitamin B-6.

Steroids A group of medications with similar chemical compositions that resemble natural anti-inflammatory agents in the body. They have many side effects including fluid retention and increasing urinary calcium.

Talwin A moderately strong pain medicine. Not an opioid.

Thiazides The name for a group of medicines that are chemically similar. They are "water pills" in that they force the kidneys to produce more urine. They are unique because they can take excess calcium in the urine and return it to the bloodstream. This is particularly beneficial in older women with high urinary calcium levels and osteoporosis.

Thiola (Alpha MPG) Used to help cystine dissolve more easily. Has fewer side effects than penicillamine.

Triamterene (Dyrenium)

A potassium sparing diuretic. Should not be used in kidney stone patients because it forms stones.

Urocit-K

An oral tablet form of potassium citrate supplement. The wax matrix tablet will often appear in the stool and some patients don't realize that the medicine has been absorbed and only the empty wax shell is expelled.

UroPhos-K

Experimental form of slow release orthophosphate. Avoids most of the side effects of orthophosphate supplements and is quite effective in calcium stone disease.

Vitamin D

The vitamin that controls intestinal absorption of calcium and phosphate from the digestive tract. Needs to be converted to its most active form, Vitamin D3, by the kidney to work. Vitamin D3 is also called calcitriol.

CHAPTER TWENTY-FIVE

Glossary

Absorptive Hypercalciuria

Abnormally high urinary calcium caused by one of several mechanisms that increase calcium absorption from the digestive tract. Type I is the most severe and doesn't respond well to dietary calcium moderation which works well in Type II. The most common cause of high urinary calcium.

Acid

Any chemical that forms chemical reactions by releasing hydrogen. In practical terms, this often destroys or digests the receiving compound depending on the strength of the acid. The most common biological acids are stomach acid and uric acid. Vinegar and lemon juice are other examples. Acids general produce a sour taste.

Acidic

Pertaining to or containing acid.

Acidosis

Condition where the body has a higher acid load than normal. Urinary citrate excretion may probably be reduced in this situation. Treatment is usually with supplemental citrate or bicarbonate.

Alkaline or Alkili

Another name for base or antacid, the opposite of acidic.

Amino Acid

One of the building blocks of protein. Formed by the combination of a carbohydrate (sugar) and a nitrogen compound.

Anaplylaxis

A severe allergic reaction in which the breathing tube or airway can swell and shut off the air supply ultimately causing death if not treated rapidly. Epinephrine (adrenalin) is the treatment of choice.

Anesthesia

Condition produced in order to permit a painless surgical operation. Loss of sensation occurs.

Anesthesiologist

A physician who specializes in the administration of anesthesia.

Balloon Dilator

An inflatable device designed to gently stretch or dilate small tubular tracts. When the injected liquid is contrast or dye, the process can be viewed by X-ray. Most often used to open the lower ureter for instrument passage, treat scarred areas of the ureter or prepare a passageway for percutaneous procedures directly on the kidney.

Base

An acid neutralizing substance such as an antacid (See Bicarbonate, Citrate).

Benign

When used in a medical context, benign means non-cancerous.

Bicarbonate

A natural form of antacid or base that is normally excreted by the pancreas to neutralize the stomach acid as your food leaves the stomach and enters the intestines. Bicarbonate is dissolved in the blood and converted to citrate by the kidneys. Common baking soda is chemically sodium bicarbonate.

Board Certified

Formal acknowledgement by a medical or surgical specialty board that the practitioner has met all requirements for specialization set by that board and has passed one or more rigorous examinations in that field. While not a guarantee of competence, it suggests a high level of knowledge in one particular specialty.

Calcitonin

A hormone made in the thyroid gland that increases calcium deposition in bone and increases urinary calcium. The opposite function to parathyroid hormone.

Calcitriol

Another name for activated Vitamin D, also called Vitamin D3.

Calcium

An important element that helps make bone and teeth hard. It's necessary for proper functioning of muscles and nerves. Normally regulated in the body primarily by the parathyroid glands. In the diet, it can be found mainly in dairy products like milk and cheese.

Calcium Oxalate

A compound made from calcium and oxalate. It can be in the monohydrate form, which is extremely hard, or dihydrate which is quite brittle. Calcium oxalate is the most frequently found ingredient in kidney stones in the United States.

Calcium Phosphate

Another compound that forms kidney stones. Calcium phosphate is more likely to occur due to a medical problem or illness. It is formed most often in alkaline solutions. There is a danger in treating some patients with uric acid stones where too much citrate or bicarbonate can alkalinize the urine too severely and allow calcium phosphate, which will not dissolve, to coat or cover the uric acid.

Calculi

The plural of calculus. Refers to many stones.

Calculus

Another name for a kidney stone. Actually, Latin for pebble or stone.

Catheter

A long, slender tube that enters the body. Most often it's used to drain the bladder but a smaller version is used for special X-rays called Retrograde Pyelograms. Catheters are flexible and usually made of latex or silicone.

Citrate

An important urinary acid neutralizer and inhibitor of kidney stone formation. It is excreted by the kidneys and will be reduced if there is too great an acid load in the body. Potassium citrate is an oral supplement available as either a liquid, tablet or dissolvable crystal packet that's used to increase the urinary citrate level.

Collecting System

The hollow, branched, interior portion of the kidney system that normally is full of urine. This is the target area for percutaneous procedures and the space in which most stones form. The exit of the collecting system (see Ureteropelvic Junction) is shaped like a funnel and leads into the ureter, the tube that connects the kidney with the urinary bladder.

Colic or Renal Colic

The extremely severe pain associated with a kidney stone attack.

Creatinine

A blood and urinary chemical that is used to estimate overall kidney function. It is produced by the muscles at a regular, predictable rate and excreted by the kidneys through simple filtration. If the blood creatinine level becomes too high, it often means that not enough blood is being filtered by the kidneys. A serum creatinine up to 1.5 to 2.0 is generally considered normal, but lower numbers are usually better.

Creatinine Clearance

A calculated value that is a good indicator of kidney function. Since serum creatinine is filtered by the kidneys based on kidney function, it is possible to measure the total urinary creatinine passed in 24 hours and calculate how much blood was filtered by the kidneys in that time to produce the creatinine found in the sample. It comes out to about 100 cc's per minute. Anything below 30 cc's is considered to be kidney failure.

Crystal

A solid form of a substance where the molecules are arranged in a repeating pattern or asymmetrical arrangement. In kidney stone disease, microscopic crystals of various stone materials can be seen in the urine when conditions are right.

CT Scan

Short for Computerized Tomography, this refers to a computer manufactured image made from a special X-ray machine. The images are very good for soft tissues but often require contrast to look into the kidneys and the intestines. Also called a "CAT" scan. Most kidney stones will show up well on CT scans.

Cystine

An amino acid or ingredient in protein. Significant because in an inherited disorder called cystinuria, very large amounts of cystine can be excreted in the urine where it can form stones. These stones tend to be difficult to treat and require life-long therapy.

Cystinuria

The presence of cystine in urine. While this does not necessarily mean an excess, when used in common language, it generally refers to abnormally high urinary levels of cystine.

Cystitis

An inflammation of the bladder which is prevalent in women. Usually caused by a urinary bladder infection.

Cystoscopy

A procedure where a special telescope, either rigid or flexible, is passed into the penis or female urethra and enters the bladder. It is used for inspection of these organs and to place tubes, ureteral catheters and Double-J stents in the ureters or kidneys.

Dehydration

The loss of excessive water from the body. Such water loss can take place through the kidneys, the lungs, or from perspiration.

Dialysis

The process in which a machine filters and cleans the blood. An artificial kidney machine.

Diuretic

Proper name for a "water pill." A medication that causes the kidney to make more urine. Often used to reduce swelling and bloating. Some diuretics have unique effects on calcium (see thiazides).

DNA

Stands for Deoxyribonucleic Acid. This is the genetic code material found in virtually every living cell. When this DNA is digested, it produces urine which ultimately forms uric acid.

Dipstick

A thin plastic strip with various chemically treated pads attached at one end. The strip with its attached pads is dipped in the urine to be tested. The various pads turns colors depending on various chemical or cellular characteristics of the urine being tested. Acid content and concentration are two of the more common tests commonly performed with urinary dipsticks. Disease specific dipsticks for kidney stone patients with identified chemical problems are under development.

Electrohydraulic Lithotripsy (EHL)

A form of kidney stone fragmentation utilizing a small electric probe. A small spark is created at the tip of the probe which is placed just next to the stone to be treated. The spark generates a small shock wave which can fragment most stones. Usually used through some type of telescope.

Enteric Hyperoxaluria

Condition usually associated with some form of chronic diarrhea and fat malabsorption. Very high levels of urinary oxalate are produced by a lack of intestinal calcium, together with chronic diarrhea and very low urinary calcium.

Extracorporeal Shock Wave Lithotripsy (ESWL)

This refers to lithotripsy, and is sometimes called ESWL. This is a large machine that generates a powerful shock wave using one of several different technologies. The generator is outside the body but the shock waves are focused at a point where the stones are located. Probably the most commonly used tool to fragment kidney stones today.

Fat Malabsorption

Condition in which fat is not digested normally leading to chronic diarrhea and excessive oxalate absorption.

Fluoroscopy

An X-ray technique where live pictures appear on a screen instead of taking a permanent picture. Used while a procedure is being done to check on progress such as trying to basket a stone. With fluoroscopy it's possible to watch the interaction between the stone and the basket. ESWL uses fluoroscopy to aim the shock waves.

French Size

Many medical tubes and catheters are measured by French Size. This represents the circumference in mm of the tube. The higher the number, the larger the tube.

Gout

A disease caused by excessively high uric acid in the blood. This high uric acid blood level will sometimes allow formation of uric acid crystals in the joints, especially at the base of the large toe. This causes intense joint pain. Can contribute to calcium and uric acid stone disease (See Gouty Diathesis). Usually treated with allopurinol when associated with kidney stones.

Gouty Diathesis

Condition in which gout is associated with uric acid or calcium oxalate kidney stone production, usually from extremely acid urine or elevated urinary uric acid excretion.

Gurney

A mobile bed with wheels designed for transport of patients in hospitals and ambulances.

Hypercalcemia

Above normal blood calcium levels. In kidney stone disease, this frequently is due to hyperparathyroidism (see below).

Hypercalciuria

Excessive urinary calcium.

Hyperoxaluria

Abnormally high urine oxalate levels.

Hyperparathyroidism

Uncontrolled, excessive secretion of the parathyroid glands, producing a disease characterized by loss of calcium from the bones. Often resulting in high serum calcium levels and kidney stones.

Hyperuricosuria

Abnormally high urinary uric acid.

Hypervitaminosis D

An uncommon condition associated with kidney stones. Caused by excessive or inappropriate Vitamin D intake.

Idiopathic

From an unknown cause.

Ileostomy

The result of intestinal surgery where the far end of the small intestine is brought out to the skin surface. The small bowel contents are then collected in a bag attached to the skin. This is normally done only for severe large bowel disease because the fluid, bicarbonate and electrolyte losses can be difficult to treat or correct, especially on a long term basis.

Intravenous (IV)

Into a vein. (For example, an intravenous medication would be injected into a vein).

Intravenous Pyelogram (IVP)

This is a series of X-rays designed to show the inside of the kidneys and urinary system. Traditionally, this was the standard diagnostic tool for evaluation of possible kidney stones and tumors. A small amount of contrast or dye is injected into a vein. This contrast is excreted by the kidneys within five to fifteen minutes. When the contrast appears in the urine, it clearly outlines the shape, size and location of the internal urinary organs. If there is blockage or dilation, it will show up clearly. Virtually all significant stones will be visible either directly on the X-ray or indirectly through the blockage they produce.

Intramuscular

An injection into the muscle. Usually abbreviated IM.

KUB

Stands for kidneys, ureters and bladder. This is just medical jargon for a flat X-ray of the abdomen. Calcium stones often show up well on this type of X-ray.

Laser

Most people now know what a laser is: a powerful, amplified beam of light that can cut through steel or tissue with ease. The laser discussed in this book is specially tuned to affect only materials that form stones. Normal tissue is not harmed. The laser is a powerful tool to fragment stones, but it requires direct contact with the stone through some sort of telescope in either the kidney, ureter or bladder.

"Lithoclast"

The proper name of a particular kidney stone fragmenting probe that uses a small version of a pneumatic hammer to fragment stones. Works very well and quite safe but relatively new and only now becoming widely available. More popular in Europe.

Lithotriptor

Literally meaning "stone breaker," it refers to any machine than can fragment a stone; usually refers to some type of ESWL machine.

Lithotripsy

The name for any procedure, surgery or technique that fragments or breaks up a stone. Often refers to ESWL.

Medullary Sponge Kidney

A benign condition of the kidneys caused by dilation of the microscopic renal collecting tubules. It's diagnosed by kidney X-rays (Intravenous Pyelogram or IVP) and is described as a faint, white blush on the inside of the kidney visible only on X-ray. It's associated with an increased risk of stone disease but isn't otherwise dangerous.

Metabolic Testing

A comprehensive package of kidney stone prevention blood and urine chemistry tests. Good commercial packages or programs are available from Laboratory Corporation of America, Mission Pharmacal, Quest Diagnostics,Urocor, Litholink and Dianon.

Metabolism

The sum total of all of the chemical reactions involved in living organisms.

Micturate

Another word for urinate or void.

"Milk Alkali" Syndrome

A condition caused by excessive oral intake of calcium containing foods and antacids.

Nephrectomy

Surgical removal of a kidney

Nephrocalcinosis

A condition where one or both kidneys is full of stones located within the renal tissue. Usually associated with an underlying medical problem like Renal Tubular Acidosis.

Nephrostomy

A surgically created passage from the skin directly into the central collecting space of the kidney. Usually a tube is left in this passage to drain the urine into a bag carried outside the body. This same passage can be enlarged and used for percutaneous procedures on the kidney.

Nephrolithiasis

Condition in which one or more stones is located in a kidney.

Nephrolithotomy

Standard surgical procedure in which the kidney is opened and a stone is removed.

Nephrologist

A medical specialist primarily in kidney problems. Nephrologists are usually involved in cases of renal failure and dialysis, but many are very interested and knowledgeable about kidney stone disease and prevention. They are not surgeons.

Nephrology

The medical specialty that deals with kidney diseases.

Nephron

The microscopic functional unit of the kidney. Each kidney is made up of thousands of nephrons.

Non-opaque

Any structure that does not show up clearly on X-ray. Most calcium containing stones would be opaque and block the X-ray beam. They would appear as white spots on standard X-ray films. A non-opaque stone would allow an X- ray beam to pass through and would be very hard to see on an X-ray film. To make it visible, some type of contrast would need to surround the non-opaque structure. The area that remained dark or clear could then be seen.

Opioid

A class of strong pain medicines derived from Opium. Morphine and Codeine would be examples.

Osteoporosis

Condition in which the bones are weak because of loss of calcium. This often occurs in people with forced immobilization, astronauts, women after menopause and in patients with hyperparathyroidism. Usually treated with supplemental calcium and either estrogen, Fosamax, calcitonin, exercise or some combination of the above.

Oxalate

A chemical compound that is found in most calcium kidney stones. It binds strongly with calcium. Dietary sources of oxalate include tea, chocolate, green leafy vegetables, nuts, tomatoes and some cola soft drinks.

Oxalobacter

The name of a normal bacteria of the intestinal tract that has the unique ability to digest oxalate. Currently used only experimentally, but has great potential as a future therapy for oxalate problems.

Parathyroid Hormone

The name of the hormone that comes from the parathyroid glands. This hormone increases blood calcium. To do this, it will increase calcium absorption from the digestive tract and take calcium away from the bones and teeth. Abnormally high levels of this hormone produce a disease called Hyperparathyroidism.

Parenteral

Means "Into the Body." Usually refers to any type of injectable medication.

PCA

Literally "Patient Controlled Analgesia." This is a program where a machine dispenses a preset amount of pain medicine directly into a vein when the patient pushes a button.

Percutaneous

Literally means through the skin. Several different types of kidney stone procedures can be done by surgically creating a passage directly into the central, open part of the kidney and passing a variety of probes, graspers, stents, catheters and other devices through the passage and into the kidney. Very useful for large or complicated stones.

pH

A measurement of the acid content of a liquid such as urine. A pH of 7 would be "neutral" like water. Acids have a low pH while alkaline liquids and bases have high pH numbers. The usual range for living organisms is between 5.0 and 9.0.

Phosphate

A normal chemical in blood and urine. Usually associated with stone disease as an inhibitor although in some stones such as calcium phosphate or struvite it can increase stone risk. One of the important chemicals to measure in any metabolic workup. Low levels of phosphate in the blood will cause an increase in Vitamin D activation and subsequent increase in intestinal absorption of phosphate and calcium.

Predisposition

The state of being particularly susceptible to a certain condition or disease.

Protease Inhibitors

A new group of medications used in the treatment of AIDS. Unfortunately, some tend to form stones.

Purine

A component of the genetic code material (DNA) inside every cell. All proteins have some purine, but the highest levels are found in red meat, poultry and fish. Digestion of excessive amounts of high purine content proteins can create high levels of uric acid.

Pyelonephritis

An infection of the kidney. Can progress to sepsis or bacterial blood poisoning.

Renal

Anything to do with the kidney.

Renal Failure

The loss of the kidneys ability to adequately filter the blood, usually due to diabetes or other diseases. When severe, requires mechanical filtration (dialysis) or kidney transplant.

Renal Leak Hypercalciuria

A type of increased urinary calcium due to a defect in the kidney that causes excessive calcium loss. Parathyroid hormone levels will tend to be elevated. This type of high urinary calcium doesn't respond to dietary modifications and requires medical therapy. Thiazides are particularly useful here. It is important never to use Cellulose therapy with renal leak hypercalciuria because it will cause a severe calcium loss.

Renal Phosphate Leak Hypercalciuria

Condition where the kidney is unable to keep excessive amounts of phosphate from being lost in the urine. This causes a low serum phosphate, high Vitamin D levels and ultimately high urinary calcium (hypercalciuria).

Renal Tubular Acidosis

Condition in which the kidneys are unable to excrete acid. It's characterized by an inability to acidify the urine even after an oral acid load. Associated with extremely low urinary citrate and severe stone disease.

Resorptive Hypercalciuria

A condition of high urinary calcium where the source of the calcium is reabsorption from existing bodily stores such as bone. Most commonly caused by hyperparathyroidism.

Retrograde Pyelogram

A special type of X-ray in which a small slender tube is placed through the bladder into the lower end of the ureter and contrast injected directly while an X-ray picture is taken. Alough this procedure requires anesthesia or sedation, the technique gives a very clear picture of the ureters and kidney interior. Can be used safely even when patients are severely allergic to contrast because there is no contact with the bloodstream.

Sepsis

A serious disease condition in which live bacteria are in the bloodstream. Can lead to an overwhelming infection and death if not treated properly and rapidly. Also called urosepsis when caused by a urinary infection.

Sodium

One of the main ingredients of table salt. Excessive salt or sodium in the diet can increase urinary calcium excretion and block the effects of some corrective medication.

Spasm

An abrupt and forceful contraction of a muscle, usually maintained for several minutes or hours and frequently associated with marked pain.

Staghorn

Refers to the branched shape of certain large stones. Usually associated with struvite or infection stones, the actual stone material can be almost any chemical stone ingredient.

Steinstrasse

Literally "street of stones." This refers to the collection of stone fragments that have lined up in the ureter and have not passed. May require additional surgery to remove. Usually happens after ESWL with large stones when a stent is not used.

Stent

A thin, slender tube designed to bypass any obstruction of the ureter such as from a stone or scar tissue. One end of the stent is placed in the kidney, and the other is in the bladder. Each end of the stent usually forms a small circle to help keep it in place. Used to help drain the kidney, bypass a stone and relieve pain. Also used as a landmark to help locate smaller or hard to see stones. Helps protect against clogging when large stones, over 1 cm in size are fragmented.

Stone Basket

One of several types of wire instruments used to capture and remove stones in the ureter. Normally used either with fluoroscopy or with special telescopes called ureteroscopes.

Stone Belt

The area of the United States where there seems to be an increased risk of kidney stones. Generally refers to the Southeast, but extends across the lower half of the country. The reason for the increased risk is only partially explained by the relatively warmer climate.

Stricture

The medical term for a narrowed or scarred area. Often occurs in the urinary system after instrumentation or stone passage. If there is a stricture of the ureter, any stones trying to pass will probably get stuck there. Stents work well to gently stretch open strictures of the ureters, but cannot help strictures of other bodily organs.

Struvite

Another name for stones caused by infection. Also called "Triple Phosphate" stones.

Tomograms

A type of X-ray where both the X-ray projector and film are revolving around the patient. This technique is able to focus better on the kidney and permit better visualization even in difficult cases. Plain tomograms without contrast will help demonstrate even relatively small stones not visible with other methods.

Triple Phosphate

Stands for magnesium, ammonium phosphate and calcium phosphate. Another name for struvite stones. The "triple" stands for the three ingredients of calcium, magnesium and ammonium that are found in these stones.

Ultrasound

High frequency sound waves. Usually used like sonar for diagnosis. Has the advantage of safety. When used as a therapeutic probe, ultrasound can drill through most stones and pulverize them.

Ureter

The name of the muscular tube that empties the kidney and carries urine down to the urinary bladder. Normally it gently squeezes the urine downwards much like the intestines slowly pass food along from the stomach to the rectum.

Ureteropelvic Junction (UPJ)

The anatomical location where the inside of the kidney connects to the ureter. It's a common place for strictures and blockages. One of the three most likely locations for a stone to get stuck.

Ureteroscope

A specially made telescope designed to be passed through the urinary bladder into the ureter. The longer, flexible versions can reach all the way up to the kidney.

Ureteroscopy

Use of the ureteroscope to examine the ureter.

Ureterovesical Junction (UVJ)

The anatomical location where the ureter joins with the urinary bladder. The entry is at an angle so that urine will not return up to the kidney during voiding when the bladder pressure is high. This is the narrowest part of the ureter and where many stones will get stuck.

Urethra

The tube that allows passage of urine from the bladder to the outside.

Uric Acid

The final chemical endpoint in humans of purine (protein) metabolism. Most of it is excreted in the urine. Uric acid can form stones, make the urine more acidic and increase calcium stone formation.

Urine

The liquid excreted by the kidneys. Normally it has a clear amber color. Urine does not normally contain sugar, albumin, pus, blood, bacteria, acetone, casts or crystals.

Urogenital Tract

The urinary and genital organs (kidney, ureter, bladder, prostate, penis, urethra, etc.).

Urinalysis

An examination of the urine. Usually best done with a chemical dipstick and a microscope, but often done just with the dipstick.

Urolithiasis

The disease process in which a stone is formed anywhere in the urinary system. While this usually refers to kidney stones, the term includes bladder stones as well.

Urology

The medical specialty field that primarily deals with surgical problems affecting the kidneys, urinary bladder and male genitalia. Urology is a surgical specialty.

Urologist

A specialist in the field of urology.

Urosepsis

A serious infection where the source of the bacteria was originally from the urinary tract.

UTI

Urinary Tract Infection. Usually refers to a bladder infection.

Vitamin D

Vitamin D is essential for absorption of calcium and phosphate particularly during childhood. It prevents rickets and helps maintain healthy teeth and bones. In excess, it can cause kidney stones. This condition is called Hypervitaminosis D.

Workup

The organized sequence of medical tests used to establish a diagnosis. A workup for diagnosis of kidney stones would include a urine examination and X-rays. A metabolic workup for stone prevention would refer to the blood and urine chemistry tests used to analyze chemical risk factors ultimately resulting in a diagnosis.

CHAPTER TWENTY-SIX

Statistically Speaking

Number of Americans affected by
kidney stones yearly .... 1.2 million

Portion of U. S. population affected annually 0.5%

Portion of population who will have
at least one kidney stone 12%

Of these, how many will have
at least one recurrence 75%

Relative risk of forming a
second stone .... 60-80% over next 10 years
(50% over next 5 years)

Rate of stone production for
recurrent stone formers .... one stone every 2-3 years

Portion of stone patients with
very aggressive disease .... 10-15% (10 or more stones)

Percentage of stone formers
who are over age 70 .... 3%

Countries with more stones
than United States .... Italy, Israel

Countries with fewer stones
than United States .... Japan, Sweden

Incidence of kidney stones in
areas of "soft" water .... Higher

Peak seasonal occurrence .... June-August

Overall incidence of kidney
stones in Japan and Sweden is .... Increasing

Overall incidence of kidney
stones in United States is .... Increasing

Who Gets Stones?

- Men get stones 3 to 4 times more often than women.
- Infection (Struvite) stones are twice as likely to occur in women as men.
- Incidence of Cystine and Uric Acid stones is about equal between the sexes.
- Caucasian people get stones 4 times more often than African-Americans.
- White-collar workers get stones more often than blue-collar workers.
- Stone attacks are most common between 20 to 40 years of age.
- Beyond age 50, risk of stone disease declines for men; increases for women.

Genetic Factors

If one family member has a stone, then the risk of another
family member developing a stone increases by 62%

Likelihood of a patient eventually forming a stone if his
brother already had one 50%

Medical Aspects

Medical problems statistically increasing risk of kidney stones:

Hyperparathyroidism, Renal Tubular Acidosis, High Blood Pressure, Arthritis, Back Pain, Chronic Diarrhea, Ileostomy, Colitis, Gout and Urinary Tract Infections

Patients with gout who will form kidney stones 25%

Stones which can be dissolved by oral
medication alone .... 5% to 10%

Number of chemicals that form kidney stones 50

Most common stone chemical
composition .... Calcium Oxalate

Proportion of stones which are calcium oxalate 70%

Stones which are visible on X-ray 90%

Stones which will pass without surgery 80%

Stones of the upper urinary tract
which will require some type of surgery 30%

Patients with "asymptomatic" stones who can expect to
eventually develop stone related problems .... >90%

Medical Evaluation and Treatment:

Expected reduction in new stone formation rate
with conservative measures only (Stone Clinic Effect) 60%

Stone patients with at least one detectable
chemical abnormality or treatable risk factor 97%

Recurrent stone patients with multiple abnormalities 85%

Patients who could expect significant reductions
in new stone formation with specific medical treatment 98%

Patients with recurrent stones who will completely stop new
stone formation while on specific medical treatment 75%

Cost Effectiveness

Number of patients annually who require
hospitalization for stones 400,000

Percentage of all hospital admissions 1%

Average cost for a hospital admission for stones $3,000

Of those patients hospitalized for stones,
proportion who will require a surgical procedure 22%

Average cost for a hospital admission for stones
when a surgical procedure is required $4500

Average cost for Extracorporeal Shock Wave
Lithotripsy (ESWL) $7500

Annual cost for stones in United States (1986) .... $2 Billion

Cost for comprehensive metabolic analysis
testing using commercial laboratory package $400

Annual net cost savings for patients with active
stone disease who have metabolic testing and
follow treatment advice. .... >$2,000

CHAPTER TWENTY-SEVEN

Stone Timeline

When was the first true operation for stones?

Probably around 50 A.D. by Celsus, a Roman physician who described an operation involving making an incision just above the rectum to enter the bladder and remove the stone.

When was the first recorded surgery for a stone?

12th Century B.C.

The Middle Ages

During this period, surgery was done primarily by barbers and was not performed even by the most reputable physicians of that period. Those who practiced other types of surgery often declined to work on urinary stones. It truly was the "Dark Ages."

Roving barbers and other "specialists" performed a variety of urinary stone procedures. Presumably they moved around a lot because if their patients survived the surgery, they probably did not live through the postoperative infections and complications.

Since stone treatment was shunned by most respectable physicians, stone surgery was therefore left to "barbers and low persons, rustics, idiots, and imbeciles, and to base and presumptuous women who are not afraid to perform it." Bruno da Langoburgo (1200 to 1286)

With the Renaissance came a new understanding of the human body and bodily functions but this occurred only slowly. The anatomical drawings and discoveries of Michelangelo and particularly Leonardo da Vinci were kept secret due to cultural prejudices of the time.

Early America

The experience of early Americans was very interesting. Urinary stone disease was, and remains, rare in Native American Indians although it remained common in the colonists. This caused some observers to mistakenly suggest that corn must be the factor that accounted for this discrepancy. Indian herbal medicines such as persimmon and sarsaparilla were adapted and used by Colonial physicians in an attempt to treat stone disease.

The Early 1500's

During the early 1500's, the "Marian Operation" for stones was developed. It included the passing of a slightly curved, smooth, solid metal probe into the bladder. When turned, the tip of the probe would encounter any bladder stones and make a clinking sound. Similar probes, called "sounds", are still used in modern urology for other purposes. The rest of the surgery was similar to that originally described by Celsus centuries earlier. An overall appraisal of the "Marian Operation" concluded that "it saved few lives and the survivors led sad lives, dripping urine, and frequently with fistulas (leaks) at the incision." Still, it was the start of the scientific approach to stone surgery.

Also during this period French surgeon, Pierre Franco, became the first surgical stone specialist. He emphasized cleanliness and wound care long before bacteria and germs were discovered. And by breaking the surgery into two stages, which allowed patients to recover somewhat from the initial incision and shock, he was able to reduce the appalling death rate from stone surgery and make it much safer. He was the first surgeon to remove a bladder stone from the "high" position, through an incision made in the lower abdomen. This approach eventually became the preferred method of removing large bladder stones in the modern era, but it would take three hundred years before most surgeons would make the change.

The first documented kidney stone surgery occurred during this period. It is credited to Cardan of Milan, who removed 18 stones from the kidney of a patient in 1550.

The Modern Era

1649   Riolan first describes a branched kidney stone that we now call a "staghorn".

1650-1780: A number of notable surgeons developed and improved on the surgical techniques of bladder stone removal. The general technique still required making an incision just above the rectum, entering the bladder and removing the stone with a forceps. Some surgeons could accomplish this feat in as little as 30 seconds. Such speed was quite important before the age of anesthesia.

1676:   Leeuwenhoek invents the microscope and discovers bacteria.

1680:   First successful, authentic open surgical removal of a stone from a kidney. However, it wasn't until the end of the 19th century that surgery directly on the kidney became an acceptable procedure. By that time, advances such as X-rays, clean technique and anesthesia had made the surgery much safer.

1682:   Francois Tolet wrote a famous textbook on surgery for stones. Helped make stone surgery an acceptable procedure that could be performed by most practicing surgeons of the time.

1731:   Academy of Surgery founded in France. Surgery started to become accepted by general public and medical practitioners as a reputable field.

1743:   Barbers were formerly forbidden to practice surgery but surgeons could no longer freely act as barbers!

1871:   First kidney surgically removed for stone disease.

1877:   Max Nitze develops the first practical telescope for looking into the bladder, called a cystoscope.

1878:   Bigelow invents mechanical instrument for crushing stones inside the bladder. It looked like a long, steel tube with an angled tip and two halves that could be separated. A screw mechanism allowed the two halves to be ground together when a stone was caught between them.

1879:   Thomas Emmet removes a stone from the ureter.

1896:   First X-ray diagnosis of a kidney stone by MacIntyre. Required 12 minutes of exposure.

1889:   First manipulation and extraction of a ureteral stone after injecting two tablespoons of sterile oil.

1906:   First retrograde pyelogram, where contrast is injected directly into the tube from the bladder to the kidney.

1911:   First removal of staghorn stone from a kidney.

1912:   Hugh Hampton Young, the "Father of Modern Urology" passed a pediatric scope through the skin directly into a massively dilated kidney. This was the first percutaneous procedure. However, it was not until the 1940's that this type of procedure was resurrected.

1923:   First intravenous pyelogram or formal kidney X-ray developed at Mayo Clinic.

1939:   Flocks is the first to make a connection between high urinary calcium and kidney stone disease.

1941:   First successful, planned percutaneous procedure to remove a stone directly from a kidney through an established passageway made from the skin.

1943:   First use of an artificial blood clot inside the kidney to help collect all the tiny stones and stone fragments during kidney surgery.

1950:   First rigid nephroscope was used to inspect the interior of a kidney during open kidney surgery. It had a 90 degree angle that allowed it to look into all the internal kidney nooks and crannies while making only a small incisional opening in the kidney itself. This instrument would be used, along with various graspers and baskets, for stone removal for the next 20 years.

1962:   First flexible ureteroscopy for stone disease performed.

1965-67:   Modern techniques for opening the collecting system of the kidney during open surgery for stones described by Gil-Vernet and Boyce. These two techniques formed the basis of contemporary open kidney surgery for stones.

1968:   Connection between gout and calcium stone disease first described. (This condition is now sometimes called "Gouty Diathesis".)

1969:   Idea for ESWL or "Stone Machine" was first discussed. Probably suggested by the physician wife of a guest at a dinner party.

1969:   Allopurinol first used for repeat calcium stone formers.

1972:   Research begins on ESWL machine in Munich, Germany.

1975:   First flexible telescope invented for stone removal by percutaneous techniques.

1978:   Enteric hyperoxaluria is described.

1980:   First patient is successfully treated by ESWL.

1983:   Importance of low urinary citrate levels in the development of recurrent calcium stones is described.

1984:   ESWL is approved by FDA and comes to the USA.

1987:   Development of first laser specifically made for kidney stone fragmentation.

1987:   First standardized commercial kidney stone prevention urine chemistry profile called "StoneRisk" is released by Mission Pharmacal.

1990:   First true "expert" computer analysis program called "CALCULUS" coupled with a comprehensive blood and urine chemistry testing protocol becomes commercially available from Laboratory Corporation of American (LabCorp).

1994:   The Kidney Stones Handbook: A Patient's Guide to Hope, Cure and Prevention" by Gail Golomb is the first book on this subject for consumers.

1999:   The second edition, updated and revised of "The Kidney Stones Handbook: A Patient's Guide to Hope, Cure and Prevention" written with Dr. Stephen w. Leslie, M.D.

2000/2001 Look for "The Kidney Stones Diet Cookbook" by Four Geez Press, and the "Stone Prevention Journal."

CHAPTER TWENTY-EIGHT

Beyond The Book— Resources

THE AMERICAN DIETETIC ASSOCIATION
216 West Jackson Blvd.
Chicago, IL 60606-6995
FAX: (312) 899-4739
Phone: (800) 877-1600
Ncndlib@eatright.org

The American Dietetic Association provides several articles published in the Journal of The American Dietetic Association. Cost per article is $15 for nonmembers and includes faxing up to 10 pages. Please include VISA or MC number and expiration date with your request.

To request a **Literature Search from the Kidney and Urologic Disease Subfile of the Combined Health Information Database (CHID)** for topics in kidney and urologic diseases contact:

NATIONAL KIDNEY AND UROLOGIC DISEASES
INFORMATION CLEARINGHOUSE
3 Information Way
Bethesda, Maryland 20892-3580
(301) 654- 4415
Fax: (301) 907-8906
e-mail: nkudic@info.niddk.nih.gov

A current list of patient education materials as well as physician-related research articles on urinary stones is available, including a free brochure *"Prevention and Treatment of Kidney Stones."*

Established in 1987, the clearinghouse provides information about diseases of the kidneys and urologic system to people with kidney and urologic disorders and to their families, health care professionals, and the public. NKUDIC answers inquiries; develops reviews and distributes publications; and works closely with professional and patient organizations and government agencies to coordinate resources about kidney and urologic diseases. Publications produced by the clearinghouse are carefully reviewed for scientific accuracy, content and readability. NIDDK is a service of the National Institute of Diabetes and Digestive and Kidney Diseases, National Institutes of Health.

THE NATIONAL KIDNEY FOUNDATION, INC.
30 East 33rd Street
New York, NY 10016
(800) 622-9010 or (212) 889-2210
http://www.kidney.org
John Davis, Executive Director

The National Kidney Foundation (NKF) mission is to prevent kidney and urinary tract diseases, improve the health and well-being of individuals and families affected by these diseases and increase the availability of organs for transplantation.

AMERICAN FOUNDATION FOR UROLOGIC DISEASE (AFUD)
1128 North Charles Street
Baltimore, MD 21201
(800) 242-2383
e-mail: admin@afud.org
http://www.afud.org

AFUD provides research grants, patient and public education and awareness, government relations and patient support group activities.

AMERICAN KIDNEY FUND (AKF)
6110 Executive Boulevard, Suite 1010
Rockville, MD 20852
(800) 638-8299 or (301) 881-3052
e-mail: helpline@akfinc.org
Fax: (301) 881-0898
http://www.arbon.com/kidney
Carol Lynn Halol, Interim Executive Director

The American Kidney Fund provides direct financial assistance, comprehensive educational programs, research grants, and community service projects for the benefit of kidney patients as well as patient and public education brochures.

AMERICAN LITHOTRIPSY SOCIETY (ALS)
70 Walnut Street
Wellesley, MA 02181
(781) 239-8203
Fax: (781) 239-7553
e-mail: prri@ix.netcom.com

This professional membership society is dedicated to addressing all aspects of lithotripsy as a treatment for both renal stones and biliary disease.

AMERICAN UROLOGICAL ASSOCIATION INC. (AUA)
1120 North Charles Street
Baltimore, MD 21201-5559
(410) 727-1100
Fax: (410) 223-4370
e-mail: aua@auanet.org
http://www.auanet.org

The AUA promotes the highest standards of urological clinical care through education, research and the formulation of health care policy. The primary professional organization for urologists.

CYSTINURIA SUPPORT NETWORK (CSN)
21001 NE 36th St.
Redmond, WA 98053
(206) 868-2996 (eve)
e-mail: cystinuria@aol.com
Jann Ledbetter, Founder

This international network provides support and an opportunity for sharing information for persons with cystinuria, a kidney disorder that causes kidney stones. Also, information, referral and newsletter.

KIDNEY FOUNDATION OF CANADA
National Office
300-5165 Sherbrooke Street West
Montreal, QC H4A 1T6

The Kidney Foundation of Canada informs Canadians about kidney disease and related disorders. This Foundation publishes a wide range of educations materials including brochures, fact sheets and a comprehensive patient manual. Good web source for kidney stone information.
http://www.kidney.ca

CROHN'S & COLITIS FOUNDATION OF AMERICA, INC.
386 Park Avenue South
17th Floor
New York, NY 10016-8804
(212) 685-3440
(800) 932-2423
FAX: (212) 779-4098
e-mail: info@ccfa.org
http://www.ccfa.org

The **National Network of Libraries of Medicine (NN/LM)**
provides health science practitioners, investigators, educators,
administrators and patients in the United States with timely,
convenient access to biomedical and health care information
resources. The network is administered by the National Library of Medicine. It consists of 8 Regional Medical Libraries,
131 Resource Libraries (primarily at medical schools) and
some 3,300 Primary Access Libraries (primarily at hospitals).
Online access to MEDLINE@ and other databases are made
available . The National Library of Medicine is part of the U.S.
Department of Health and Human Services, Public Health
Service of the National Institutes of Health in Bethesda, Maryland 20894. Each regional Library will direct you to a medical
library or libraries closest to your home.

The following is a list of the **Regional Medical Libraries** and
the areas served by each.

MIDDLE ATLANTIC REGION
The New York Academy of Medicine
2 East 103rd Street
New York, New York 10029
(212) 876-8763
(212) 534-7042 (Fax)
States served: Delaware, New Jersey, New York, Pennsylvania

SOUTHEASTERN/ATLANTIC REGION
University of Maryland at Baltimore
Health Sciences Library
111 South Greene Street
Baltimore, Maryland 21201-1583
(301) 328-0099
(301) 328-0099
States served: Alabama, Florida, Georgia, Maryland, Mississippi, North Carolina, South Carolina, Tennessee, Virginia, West Virginia, the District of Columbia, Puerto Rico, and the U.S. Virgin Islands

GREATER MIDWEST REGION
University of Illinois at Chicago
Library of the Health Sciences
P.O. Box 7509
Chicago, Illinois 60680
(312) 996-2464
(312) 996-2226 (fax)
States served: Iowa, Illinois, Indiana, Kentucky, Michigan, Minnesota, North Dakota, Ohio, South Dakota, and Wisconsin

MIDCONTINENTAL REGION
University of Nebraska Medical Center
Leon S. McGoogan Library of Medicine
600 South 42nd Street
Omaha, Nebraska 68198-6706
(402) 559-4326
(402) 559-5498 (Fax)
States served: Colorado, Kansas, Missouri, Nebraska, Utah, and Wyoming

SOUTH CENTRAL REGION
Houston Academy of Medicine-Texas Medical Center Library
1133 M.D. Anderson Boulevard
Houston, Texas 77030
(713) 790-7053
(713) 790-7030 (Fax)
States served: Arkansas, Louisiana, New Mexico, Oklahoma, and Texas

PACIFIC NORTHWEST REGION
University of Washington
Health Sciences Center Library, SB-55
Seattle, Washington 98195
(206) 543-8262
(206) 543-2469 (Fax)
States served: Alaska, Idaho, Montana, Oregon, and Washington

PACIFIC SOUTHWEST REGION
University of California at Los Angeles
Louise Darling Biomedical Library
10833 Le Conte Avenue
Los Angeles, California 90024-1798
(213) 825-1200
(213) 825-5389
States served: Arizona, California, Hawaii, Nevada, and U.S.
Territories in the Pacific Basin

NEW ENGLAND REGION
University of Connecticut Health Center
Lyman Maynard Stowe Library
263 Farmington Avenue
Farmington, Connecticut 06034-4003
(203) 679-4500
(203) 679-4046
States served: Connecticut, Maine, Massachusetts, New
Hampshire, Rhode Island, and Vermont

For more information about specific Network programs in
your region, call the Regional Medical Library in your area at
their direct number or dial 1-800-338-7657. This number is a
toll-free line for all Regional Medical Libraries.

For general Network information contact:
National Network of Libraries of Medicine
National Library of Medicine
8600 Rockville Pike
Building 38, Room B1-E03
Bethesda, MD 20894
(301) 496-4777

OXALOSIS AND HYPEROXALURIA FOUNDATION **(OHF)**
12 Pleasant Street
Maynard, MA 01754
(888) 712-2432, pin # 5392, or (508) 461- 0614
e-mail: exec-dir@ohf.org
http://www.ohf.org
Tammy Murphy, Executive Director

OHF assists in informing the public, especially patients,
parents, families, physicians and medical professionals about
hyperoxaluria and related condition., ie., oxalosis and calcium-
oxalate kidney stones, provides a support network for those
affected by hyperoxaluria, and supports and encourages
research to find a cure for hyperoxaluria.

POLYCYSTIC KIDNEY RESEARCH FOUNDATION
4901 Main Street, Suite 200
Kansas City, MO 64112-2634
(800) PKD-CURE or (816) 931-2600
Fax: (816) 931-8655
e-mail: pkdcure@pkrfoundation.org
Dan Larson, President
Tanja Heinen, Vice President

This Foundation promotes research in the cause and cure of
polycystic kidney disease. A patient manual "Polycystic
Kidney Disease" quarterly newsletter (PKR Progress) and
other materials are available.

SOCIETY OF UROLOGIC NURSES AND ASSOCIATES **(SUNA)**
East Holly Avenue
Box 56
Pitman, NJ 08071-0056
(609) 256-2335
Fax: (609) 589-7463
e-mail: suna@mail.ajj.com
http://www.inurse.com/-SUNA
Ron Brady, Executive Director

SUNA is a professional organization of urologic nurses com-
mitted to excellence in patient care standards and a continuum
of quality care, clinical practice, and research through education of its members, patients, family and community.

For Information on Your Medical Records

For a copy of the 69-page booklet *Medical Records: Getting Yours,* which provides information and advice on obtaining your medical records and includes a state-by- state survey of the laws governing patient access: Send $10 to Public Citizen's Health Research Group, Publications Manager, Dept. MR2, 2000 P St. NW, Ste 700, Washington, DC 20036.

For a copy of your Medical Information Bureau record (if one exists): contact MIB Information Office, PO Box 105, Essex Station, Boston, MA 02112 (617) 426-3660); Canadian residents contact MIB at 330 University Ave., Ste 102, Toronto, Ontario, Canada M5G 1R7 (416) 597-0590. If you find an error you can ask MIB to correct it.

A free brochure on "Your Health Information Belongs to You" is available through the American Health Information Management Association (AHIMA), Professional Practice Division, 919 N. Michigan Avenue, Suite 1400, Chicago, IL 60611. The phone number is (800) 621-6828

Recommended Books

Oxalate Content of Selected Foods with Recipes and Menu Suggestions, Second Edition
The General Clinical Research Center, UC San Diego Medical Center, 9500 Gilman Drive, La Jolla, CA 92093-0008
Phone: 1-800-520-7323, FAX: (619) 822-0216
$12, includes shipping and handling. Calif. residents, please add 7.25% sales tax.

Milk is Not for Every Body: Living with Lactose Intolerance
Steve Carper
Penguin Books, 375 Hudson Street, New York, NY 10014
ISBN: 0-452-27711-6
USA $13.95, CAN $ 17.99

Irritable Bowel Syndrome & Diverticulosis: A Self-Help Plan
Shirley Trickett
HarperCollins Publishers, 77-85 Fulham Palace Road, Hammersmith, London W6 8JB or 1160 Battery Street, San Francisco, California 94111-1213
ISBN: 0-7225-2401-3
USA $11.00, CAN $11.95

Your Body's Many Cries for Water
F. Batmanghelidj, M.D.
Global Health Solutions, Inc., P.O. Box 3189, Falls Church, VA
22043, (703) 848-2333, (703) 848-2334 (FAX)
ISBN: 0-962994-3-2-5
$14.95, plus S/H $3.00

You Don't Have to Live with Cystitis
Larrian Gillespie, M.D.
Avon Books
Healthy Life Publications , 264 South La Cienega Blvd.,
PMB #1233, Beverly Hills, CA 90211, (801) 760-2384
FAX 1-800-554-3335
e-mail: lgille01@interserv.com, web site: menopausediet.com
ISBN: 0-380-78779-2
This book is available from bookstores nationwide.
Also, great resource for books on menopause.

What do kidney stones look like? For actual color photos from
one of the most informative web sites on the chemical composition of kidney stones, visit the friendly folks at Louis C.
Herring Laboratory and Company. This laboratory analyzes
the chemical make-up of kidney stones (maybe they analyzed
yours?). The web site has interesting facts about stones. Visit
http://www.herringlab.com.

To contact Gail Savitz or Stephen W. Leslie, M.D.:
Visit our web page at:
http://www.readersndex.com/fourgeez
or
e-mail: ggolomb@ns.net or phone: (800) 2-KIDNEYS

Index

C

caffeine 84, 128, 131, 135, 137, 179
Calcibind 87
calcitriol 76, 226, 231, 235
calcium 29-30, 62, 67, 69, 73, 76-80, 82-83, 85-90, 93-99, 103, 116, 119, 138, 141, 181, 182, 184-186, 190, 191, 194, 199, 200, 203, 216, 217, 219, 221, 225, 226, 228, 230, 231, 235, 238, 239, 240, 241, 242, 243, 244, 245, 246, 248, 249, 250, 259, 268
  Calcium Information Center 178
  Calcium Loading Test 73, 74, 87
  citrate 31, 61, 62, 67, 70, 71, 72, 82, 86, 88, 90, 92, 98, 99, 100, 103, 107, 115, 116, 119, 136, 139, 142, 182, 205, 219, 226, 229, 233, 234, 235, 236
  hyperabsorption 87, 93, 178, 179
  loss 78, 87, 179, 246
  metabolism 114
  oxalate 31, 35, 61, 62, 65, 67, 69, 72, 83, 86, 89, 90, 95, 98-103, 139, 175, 185, 204, 228, 235
  phosphate 68, 71, 76, 77, 80, 90, 91, 98, 121, 139, 146, 147, 148, 235, 245, 248
  supplement 73, 99, 113, 114-116, 119, 205, 226
catheters 78, 82-83, 122, 123, 237, 239, 244
cellulose 74-75, 84, 87, 89, 226, 246
chemotherapy 67, 72, 203
children
  Lasix 203
  Metabolic problems 202
  stone prevention 204-205,
  therapy 204
cholestyramine 99-100, 103, 226
Citrolith 90
Coca-Cola® 136, 177
Coe, Fredric L., M.D. 105, 178, 212
colchicine 204
colic 53, 106, 202, 213-215, 236
colitis 29, 32, 97, 253, 265

contrast agent 55
coronary artery disease 113
cranberry juice 127, 128
creatinine level 26, 28, 236
Crohn's disease 29, 32, 97
crystal 25, 31, 32, 46, 47, 68, 71, 83, 86, 92, 99, 100, 132, 133, 147, 167, 203, 220, 229, 236, 237, 239, 249
crystal formation 90, 97, 100
CT Scans 20, 21, 34, 48, 54, 56, 57, 69, 237
Cuprimine 149
Curhan, Gary, M.D. 115, 139, 177
cystic fibrosis 204
cystine 29, 33, 145-150, 226, 230, 252
cystinuria 33, 145-150, 200, 202, 227, 229, 237, 264
Cystinuria Support Network 150, 264
cystitis
  32, 100, 130, 227, 237, 284.
  See UTI
cystoscopy 56

D

Davis, Adelle 182
degenerative diseases 28
dehydration 29, 32, 49, 69, 83, 93, 97, 100, 131, 133, 137, 144, 238
Demerol 41, 42, 43, 227
diabetes 28, 55, 113, 245, 262
dialysis 26, 28, 238, 243, 245
Diamox 90, 148, 227
Dianon 109, 111, 242
diarrhea, chronic 29, 32, 69, 88, 90, 96, 97, 98, 99, 106, 238, 239, 253
diet, high carbohydrate 84
diet, low calcium 73, 74, 75, 96, 115
diet protein 36, 84, 86, 96, 97
diet, vegetarian 36, 148, 183
diet therapy 66, 175, 200
dietary measures 30, 74, 84, 86, 87, 101, 182
dietary modifications 59, 87, 246

Send a Copy of This Book
to a Friend

You may know a person or two, among all your friends and relatives, who is in need of information found in this book. Someone who could benefit and appreciate receiving a copy.

For additional copies we suggest you first try your local bookstores. But, if they happen to be out of stock, we will be pleased to receive your order directly, and it will be shipped immediately. Just drop a letter with your name and address, and check or money order for each book purchased. The price is $17.95 plus $3.20 postage and handling (California residents add $1.30 sales tax).

Send to:

Four Geez Press
PMB 131, 1911 Douglas Blvd., Suite 85
Roseville, CA 95661

☐ **Yes!** *Please send me my copy of THE KIDNEY STONES HANDBOOK. Enclosed is a check or money order in the amount of $17.95 plus $3.20 shipping.*

Ship To _____

Name _____

City _____

State _____ Zip _____

Daytime phone _____

I prefer to charge my credit card ☐ *VISA* ☐ MASTERCARD

Card number _____

Exp. Date _____

Signature _____

California residents please add $1.30 sales tax. Mail to:
Four Geez Press, PMB 131, 1911 Douglas Blvd., Suite 85, Roseville, CA 95661

✂ - - - - - - - - - - - ✂ - - - - - - - - - - - ✂

☐ **Yes!** *Please send me my copy of THE KIDNEY STONES HANDBOOK. Enclosed is a check or money order in the amount of $17.95 plus $3.20 shipping.*

Name _____

Address _____

City _____

State _____ Zip _____

Daytime phone _____

I prefer to charge my credit card ☐ *VISA* ☐ MASTERCARD

Card number _____

Exp. Date _____

Signature _____

California residents please add $1.30 sales tax. Mail to:
Four Geez Press, PMB 131, 1911 Douglas Blvd., Suite 85, Roseville, CA 95661

Gail Savitz entered medical reporting shortly after graduation from California State University Long Beach. When stricken twice with kidney stones in 1991, and discovering very little consumer information available, she used her painful experiences, extensive research, and journalism background to write this book. She has been free of any new kidney 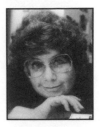 stones since she began practicing the stone prevention tips and suggestions that eventually became the basis for The Kidney Stones Handbook. Savitz is a member of the American Medical Writers Association. She is also the editor of the Kidney Stones Network Newsletter, a quarterly publication for stone patients who want to know about the latest research and recommendations for kidney stone disease prevention.

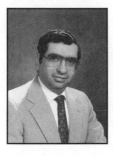 **Stephen W. Leslie, M.D., F.A.C.S.**, a board certified urologist specializing in the diagnosis and treatment of kidney stone disease, is an Assistant Clinical Professor of Urology at the Medical College of Ohio School of Medicine, and Physician Affiliate of the Cleveland Clinic. He is the Founder and Medical Director of the Lorain Kidney Stone Research Center and the developer of the "CALCULUS" kidney stone prevention program which won the prestigious "Thirlby Award" of the American Urological Association. Dr. Leslie is working with Gary Curhan, M.D., of Harvard University in ongoing kidney stone disease research and prevention. Dr. Leslie serves as Editor-In-Chief of the EMEDICINE.COM Urology Medical Textbook which has been authorized by the National Library of Medicine to serve as the authoritative Internet medical reference source for health care professionals. He has written and published over a hundred articles for various medical publications and for the lay reader on urologic and medical issues.